D1509468

Review of Perioperative Nursing

Bettyann Hutchisson, R.N., B.S.N., C.N.O.R.
Nurse Clinician, Perioperative Education
The Methodist Hospital
Houston, Texas

Mark L. Phippen, R.N., M.N., C.N.O.R.
Clinical Educator
Valleylab, Inc.
Boulder, Colorado

Maryann Papanier Wells, Ph.D., R.N., C.N.O.R., F.A.A.N.
Nurse Manager, Perioperative Nursing
The Hospital of the University of Pennsylvania
Philadelphia, Pennsylvania

Review of Perioperative Nursing

W.B. SAUNDERS COMPANY
A Harcourt Health Sciences Company
Philadelphia   London   Toronto   Sydney

Mohawk Valley Community College Library

W.B. SAUNDERS COMPANY
A Harcourt Health Sciences Company

The Curtis Center
Independence Square West
Philadelphia, Pennsylvania 19106

Editor: Thomas Eoyang
Designer: Ellen Zanolle
Production Manager: Frank Polizzano
Manuscript Editor: Tina Rebane
Cover Designer: Ellen Zanolle

Library of Congress Cataloging-in-Publication Data

Hutchisson, Bettyann.

   Review of perioperative nursing/Bettyann Hutchisson, Mark L. Phippen, Maryann Papanier Wells.

   p.; cm.

  ISBN 0–7216–3413–3

   1. Operating room nursing—Examinations, questions, etc. I. Title: Perioperative nursing. II. Phippen, Mark L. III. Wells, Maryann M. Papanier. IV. Title.

  [DNLM: 1. Perioperative Nursing—Examination Questions. WY 18.2 H978r 2000]

RD32.3.H88 2000

610.73′677′076—dc21   99-051714

REVIEW OF PERIOPERATIVE NURSING   ISBN 0–7216–3413–3

Copyright © 2000 by W.B. Saunders Company.

All rights reserved. No part of this publication may be reproduced or transmitted in any form or by any means, electronic or mechanical, including photocopy, recording, or any information storage and retrieval system, without permission in writing from the publisher.

Printed in the United States of America.

Last digit is the print number: 9   8   7   6   5   4   3   2   1

RD
32.3
.H88
2 000

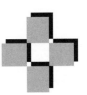

Contributing Authors

Cheri Ackert-Burr, M.S.N., Ba.Ed., R.N., C.N.O.R.
Advanced Sterilization Products, A Division of Johnson & Johnson Medical, Inc.,
Kingwood, Texas
Handling Tissues with Instruments

Mary V. "Ginny" Baird, R.N., C.N.O.R.
Nurse Clinician, Perioperative Education, Methodist Healthcare System, Houston, Texas
Positioning the Patient

Ellen L. (Burns) Creakbaum, R.N., C., M.S.
Nursing Program Specialist, Methodist Healthcare System, Houston, Texas
Facilitating Care After the Operative or Invasive Procedure

Anney Schneweis, R.N.
Patient Care Coordinator, Post Anesthesia Care Unit (PACU), Methodist Healthcare
System, Houston, Texas
Physiologically Monitoring the Patient

Rosemarie Wheeler, R.N., C.N.O.R.
Staff Nurse, Operating Room, Methodist Healthcare System, Houston, Texas
Providing Hemostasis

Preface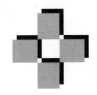

Review of Perioperative Nursing was written for nurses interested in validating their knowledge concerning the practice of perioperative nursing. This book is composed of fifteen chapters that address multiple facets of perioperative nursing, from creating and maintaining a sterile field to caring for the patient following the procedure. Each chapter begins with a brief introduction and then provides a series of test questions concerning the chapter topic. Over 700 questions for this book were developed using Phippen and Wells's *Patient Care During Operative and Invasive Procedures* as a reference. At the end of each chapter, answers with rationales are provided for each question.

Bettyann Hutchisson
Mark L. Phippen
Maryann P. Wells

NOTICE

Nursing is an ever-changing field. Standard safety precautions must be followed, but as new research and clinical experience broaden our knowledge, changes in treatment and drug therapy become necessary or appropriate. Readers are advised to check the product information currently provided by the manufacturer of each drug to be administered to verify the recommended dose, the method and duration of administration, and the contraindications. It is the responsibility of the treating physician, relying on experience and knowledge of the patient, to determine dosages and the best treatment for the patient. Neither the publisher nor the editor assumes any responsibility for any injury and/or damage to persons or property.

THE PUBLISHER

Contents

Chapter 1
Preparation of the Patient for the Procedure: Legal and Ethical Considerations   1

Chapter 2
Preparation of the Patient for the Procedure: Physical, Psychological, and Emotional Considerations   7

Chapter 3
Transferring the Patient   17

Chapter 4
Assisting the Anesthesia Provider   27

Chapter 5
Establishing and Maintaining a Sterile Field   35

Chapter 6
Performing Sponge, Sharp, and Instrument Counts   47

Chapter 7
Providing Instruments, Equipment, and Supplies   55

Chapter 8
Administering Drugs and Solutions   71

Chapter 9
Physiologically Monitoring the Patient   83

Chapter 10
Monitoring and Controlling the Environment   91

Chapter 11
Positioning the Patient   105

Chapter 12
Handling Cultures and Specimens   121

Chapter 13
Handling Tissues With Instruments   129

Chapter 14
Providing Hemostasis   143

Chapter 15
Facilitating Care After the Operative or Invasive Procedure   155

CHAPTER 1

Preparation of the Patient for the Procedure: Legal and Ethical Considerations

The legal and ethical rights of patients are primary concerns for professional nurses providing care during operative and invasive procedures. In their role as patient advocates, nurses may be called on to protect the rights of patients who lack the ability to act on their own behalf. In their role as patient educators, nurses inform patients of their legal and ethical rights related to operative and invasive procedure care. The questions for this chapter will help the reader assess his or her knowledge about

• Autonomy and authorization for
  treatment
• Nonmaleficence and malpractice

The reference used for this chapter is Phippen, M. L., & Wells, M. P. (1999). *Patient care during operative and invasive procedures.* Philadelphia: W. B. Saunders, pp. 13–16.

Questions

1. The best way to deal with legal issues in the operative and invasive procedure period is:

   a. Good communication techniques

   b. Excellent legal counsel

   c. Patient and family involvement in patient care

   d. Good physician and nurse relationship

2. The ethical principle of autonomy is also legally recognized as:

   a. Affirmative duty

   b. Right to informed consent

   c. Prima facie

   d. Beneficence

3. The legal obligation to provide the information and obtain the consent in the case of operative and invasive procedures lies with the:

   a. Circulating nurse

   b. Physician

   c. Hospital administrator

   d. Unit nurse

4. Mr. Smith has been admitted to the preoperative holding area. During the assessment the nurses discovers that Mr. Smith does not understand the risks associated with the operative procedure he is about to undergo. What is the appropriate action for the nurse to take?

   a. Reschedule the procedure for the next day

   b. Explain the risks to the patient

   c. Notify the physician

   d. Have Mr. Smith sign the consent form anyway

5. When should the process of documenting the patient's consent take place?

   a. Immediately before the operative procedure

   b. After the patient is admitted to the hospital for the procedure

   c. In the physician's office a few days before the operative procedure

d. At the time the physician identifies the patient in the operative procedure suite

6. Mechanisms created by state statutes to legally protect the patient's ethical right to self-determination are known as:

   a. Informed consent

   b. Nonmaleficence

   c. American Nurses Association (ANA) code for nurses

   d. Advance directives

7. Living wills and durable power of attorney are examples of:

   a. Advance directives

   b. Standards of nursing care

   c. Association of Operating Room Nurses (AORN) recommendations for nursing activities

   d. Guidelines for physician activities

8. How long is a patient's consent or refusal of treatment considered valid?

   a. Forever

   b. The length of the hospital admission

   c. As long as circumstances underlying the decision remain unchanged

   d. Until the patient contacts a lawyer to make changes to the document

9. When does the law "assume consent" for an operative or invasive procedure?

   a. Never

   b. When the patient's condition is such that consent cannot be obtained but the procedure is one for which a reasonable person would grant consent

   c. When the patient is not of legal age and the parent or guardian cannot be found

d. When the patient suffers from a mental disorder that does not allow freedom of choice

10. The ethical tenet that a person does not harm other persons or himself or herself is known as:

    a. Contributory negligence

    b. Beneficence

    c. Malpractice

    d. Nonmaleficence

11. What does negligence law allow?

    a. Patients to sue for compensation for injuries

    b. Physicians' safety from lawsuits

    c. Captain-of-the-ship lawsuits

    d. Patients' arrangement for someone to speak on their behalf

12. How is legal duty enforced?

    a. Principles of beneficence

    b. ANA standard of care

    c. Negligence law

    d. Principles of nonmaleficence

13. What is the most common action that results in successful suits against nurses?

    a. Incorrect consent forms

    b. Retained foreign body

    c. Sterilization issues

    d. Prolonged surgical procedures

14. What can the nurse do to prevent the patient from receiving injuries during the operative or invasive procedure, which will decrease the number of lawsuits filed against nurses?

    a. Perform preoperative assessment

    b. Include the family in nursing care

c. Allow patient to make all decisions about care

d. Have good working relationship with physician

15. Nurses cannot meet legal and ethical duties for safe patient care in the ambulatory setting without the aid of:

a. Comprehensive patient-teaching programs

b. Advanced nursing degrees

c. Physician participation in home-going instruction

d. ANA standard of care

16. In the ambulatory setting, when should the patient make arrangements to have someone else drive him or her home after the procedure?

a. Before being discharged from the hospital

b. Before preoperative medications have been given

c. At the time the procedure was scheduled

d. At the time the decision was made to have the procedure

17. What is contributory negligence?

a. The hospital will not do the patient harm

b. Captain-of-the-ship standard

c. Nurse must be reasonable and prudent

d. Patient must be reasonable and prudent

18. To be most effective, teaching materials should be:

a. Handwritten

b. In the language of the patient

c. Mailed to the patient before the procedure

d. Explained by the physician

19. When should patient preparation for an operative or invasive procedure begin?

a. When the patient is admitted to the hospital

b. Before preoperative medication is given

c. During the initial decision to have an operative or invasive procedure

d. At the time of scheduling of the operative or invasive procedure

❖ Answers

1. [a] Good communication techniques

Most of the difficult legal and ethical issues that can arise during the operative and invasive procedure period are best dealt with through good communication and preparation of the patient. Patients and their families or caregivers who receive information before the procedure are better able to actively participate in the planning and decision-making process. (*page 13*)

2. [b] Right to informed consent

The ethical principle of autonomy is also legally recognized as a right to informed consent. The right of patients to be free of procedures to which they did not consent was recognized as early as 1914 in the landmark care of *Schloendorf v Society of New York Hospital (1914.)* (*page 13*)

3. [b] Physician

It is well established that the legal obligation to provide the information and obtain the consent lies with the person performing the procedure—namely, the physician—in the case of operative and invasive procedures. (*page 13*)

4. [c] Notify the physician

If the patient has not discussed the procedure with the physician or if the patient is requesting information related to the medical nature of the procedure, such as its risks, benefits, and alternatives, those questions should be referred to the physician. (*page 13*)

5. [c] In the physician's office a few days before the operative procedure

It is far preferable that the process of documenting the patient's consent take place well in advance of transporting the patient to the procedure room. This allows for clarification of any needed information without interference from time pressure or medications. (*page 14*)

6. [d] Advance directives

A newer area of the law that is developing to legally protect the patient's ethical right to autonomy and self-determination is that of advance directives. These are mechanisms created by state statutes (products of the legislatures). (*page 14*)

7. [a] Advance directives

Living wills and durable power of attorney for healthcare are two prevalent examples of advance directives. (*page 14*)

8. [c] As long as the circumstance underlying the decision remain unchanged

A patient's consent or refusal of treatment is considered valid as long as the circumstances underlying the decision remain unchanged, that is, as long as the risks, benefits, and alternatives are the same. (*page 14*)

9. [b] When the patient's condition is such that consent cannot be obtained but the procedure is one for which a reasonable person would grant consent

When the patient's condition is such that consent cannot be obtained and the procedure is one that a reasonable person would likely consent to, the law will assume consent. This position is consistent with the ethical principle of beneficence. (*page 15*)

10. [d] Nonmaleficence

The ethical principles of nonmaleficence (literally, to not do harm) hold that an ethical person does not harm other persons or himself or herself. (*page 15*)

11. [a] Patients to sue for compensation for injury

Negligence law allows a patient to sue for compensation for injuries that are caused (or that are not prevented) by the unreasonable action or inaction of another. (*page 15*)

12. [c] Negligence law

Legal duty is the action of conducting oneself as a reasonable and prudent professional and not causing injury to patients. This legal duty is enforced through negligence law and malpractice law. (*page 15*)

13. [b] Retained foreign body

The most common actions or omissions that have resulted in successful suits against nurses providing care during operative and invasive procedures involve retained foreign bodies, medication errors, positioning errors, improper use of equipment, and the nurse's inattention to the patient's condition. (*page 15*)

14. [a] Perform preoperative assessment

Many patient injuries can be prevented through good assessment and preparation of the patient before the procedure. For example, nurses' long-standing practices of assessing the patient before the procedure for allergies, mobility, skin condition, body size, and so forth, enable better planning and interventions to prevent injuries. (*page 15*)

15. [a] Comprehensive patient-teaching programs

The nurse cannot meet his or her legal and ethical duties of safe patient care in the ambulatory setting without comprehensive patient-teaching programs. The patient and lay caregivers must know how to perform safe care: what to watch for, what to do, and when and how to seek additional attention. (*page 15*)

16. [c] At the time the procedure was scheduled

Patients must know ahead of time they cannot drive themselves home after the procedure. This preparation should begin when the procedure is scheduled so that arrangements can be made; it cannot wait until the morning of the procedure. (*page 15*)

17. [d] Patient must be reasonable and prudent

Contributory negligence is another component of negligence law. It requires that patients be reasonable and prudent. Patients who have not followed instructions can be denied compensation even if they would otherwise have had a successful suit. (*page 15*)

18. [b] In the language of the patient

To be most effective—as evidence in a contributory negligence defense and as teaching tools—teaching materials should be written in a manner appropriate to the reading level and language of the patient and should be discussed with the patient and the accompanying caregiver. (*page 16*)

19. [c] During the initial decision to have an operative or invasive procedure

For the physician and patient, preparation begins during the initial decision making about the prospect of an operative or invasive procedure. For nurses caring for patients undergoing operative and invasive procedures, preparation begins no later than the time of scheduling. (*page 16*)

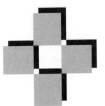

CHAPTER 2

Preparation of the Patient for the Procedure: Physical, Psychological, and Emotional Considerations

Preparing the patient for the procedure refers to the activities done by the registered nurse before the operative or invasive procedure to make the patient physically, psychologically, and emotionally ready for the procedure. The questions for this chapter will help the reader assess his or her knowledge about

- Facilitating patient admission to the healthcare facility
- Identifying existing alterations in health status that contribute to the patient's risk for adverse outcomes before, during, and after the operative or invasive procedure
- Facilitating preprocedure care

The reference used for this chapter is Phippen, M. L., & Wells, M. P. (1999). *Patient care during operative and invasive procedures.* Philadelphia: W. B. Saunders, pp. 17–41.

✚ Questions

1. What does the nurse use to diagnose actual or potential alterations in health that may affect the patient during the operative or invasive procedure period?

   a. Laboratory studies

   b. Physical examination

   c. Patient assessment

   d. Operative history

2. The physician uses the assessment data to:

   a. Establish the patient's risk of postprocedure complications

   b. Diagnose potential alterations in health that may affect the patient during the procedure

   c. Facilitate the admission process before the operative procedure

   d. Establish rapport and put the patient at ease during the preprocedure period

3. What is the purpose of shaking the patient's hand during the introduction?

   a. Assists with diagnostic procedures

   b. Defines who is in charge of the interview

   c. Facilitates the interview process

   d. Establishes rapport

4. How should the nurse begin the patient assessment?

   a. Take vital signs

   b. Explain the operative procedure

   c. Introduce oneself

   d. Discuss the risks associated with the operative procedure

5. On June 20, 1999, Allen Walters was admitted to the hospital for an inguinal hernia repair. He was born on July 24, 1997. How will the nurse record his chronological age?

   a. 23 months

   b. 1 year 11 months

   c. 2 years

   d. DOB: 7-24-97

6. Why is it important to have the patient's accurate weight on the chart?

   a. Proper calculation of medications

   b. Identification of potential positioning problems

   c. If abnormal, a nutritional consult can be requested

   d. Discussion of potential risks from anesthesia

7. Judy Bowers' preoperative vital signs are as follows: temperature 98.8°F, pulse 132 beats/min, respirations 16 breaths/min, and blood pressure 172/94. The postoperative complication the nurse will be looking for is:

   a. Fluid imbalance

   b. Infection

   c. Renal failure

   d. Atelectasis

8. Normal respirations on an adult would be:

   a. Less than 10 breaths/min

   b. 12–18 breaths/min

   c. 18–24 breaths/min

   d. More than 24 breaths/min

9. A possible indication for an abnormal finding of bradypnea is:

   a. Pain

   b. Infection

   c. Anemia

   d. Brain lesion

10. An abnormal finding of hypertension can lead to the postoperative complication of:

    a. Atelectasis

    b. Vascular collapse

    c. Increased intracranial pressure

    d. Hemorrhage

11. What blood study result would alert the perioperative nurse to an unsuspected inflammatory process in a patient who has undergone an operative or invasive procedure?

    a. Chloride level of 88 mEq/L

    b. White blood cell count of 17,000 cells/mm

    c. Blood urea nitrogen level of 8 mg/dL

    d. Sodium level of 130 mEq/L

12. Zachary Hall has been scheduled for emergency surgery for gastrointestinal bleeding. What blood study will assist in determining the need for blood replacement before the procedure?

    a. Prothrombin time

    b. Creatinine

    c. Potassium

    d. Hematocrit

13. A potassium level of 5.9 mEq/L could indicate:

    a. Excessive use of diuretics

    b. Dehydration

    c. Hypotension

    d. Malnutrition

14. A carbon dioxide level of 20 mEq/L could indicate:

    a. Respiratory acidosis

    b. Hyperventilation

    c. Intestinal obstruction

    d. Chronic obstructive pulmonary disease

15. What does a low white blood cell count indicate?

    a. Bone marrow depression

    b. Infection

    c. Gastrointestinal bleeding

    d. Liver failure

16. An increase in blood urea nitrogen is indicative of:

   a. Overhydration

   b. Liver damage

   c. Dehydration

   d. Malnutrition

17. A serological study will determine:

   a. Presence of syphilis

   b. Vaginal tumors

   c. Diabetic acidosis

   d. Casts in the urine

18. The presence of syphilis is determined by a serological study. What other determinations will a serological study show?

   a. Infectious mononucleosis

   b. Diabetes insipidus

   c. Adrenal insufficiency

   d. Hyperaldosteronism

19. Dark amber urine indicates:

   a. Blood in the urine

   b. Infection

   c. Glomerular disorders

   d. Concentrated urine

20. Bill Wheeler is scheduled for a total knee replacement of the right knee. He is 38 years old and has a history of coronary artery disease. The nurse will check the chart for what test?

   a. Serological studies

   b. 12-Lead electrocardiogram (ECG)

   c. Normal ECG

   d. Chest radiography

21. The physical examination reveals skin tissue on the right leg that appears shiny, taut, and paler than the rest of the body. This leg would be considered to have:

   a. A primary lesion

   b. An allergy

   c. Edematous tissue

   d. A secondary lesion

22. What causes dependent edema?

   a. Endocrine imbalance

   b. Fluid volume deficit

   c. Latex allergies

   d. Cardiac insufficiency

23. If the patient is an ambulatory patient, where is pitting edema most commonly found?

   a. Dorsum of the foot

   b. Sacrum

   c. Buttocks

   d. Lower back

24. What would cause nonpitting edema?

   a. Electrolyte imbalance

   b. Inflammatory responses

   c. Endocrine imbalance

   d. The aging process

25. In skin assessment, a yellow-orange color may indicate:

   a. Increased blood flow to the skin

   b. Increased serum carotene level

   c. Endocrine imbalance

   d. Autonomic nervous system stimulation

26. If the nurse is able to percuss the apex of the heart past the midclavicular line, it is an indication of:

    a. Cardiomegaly

    b. Early arteriosclerosis

    c. Respiratory failure

    d. Normal findings

27. Diffuse yellow to brown nail beds are an indication for:

    a. Jaundice

    b. Chronic hepatic disease

    c. Cardiac insufficiency

    d. Trichinosis

28. A vertical brown banding extending from the proximal nail fold distally is indicative of:

    a. Shock

    b. Diabetes

    c. Normal aging

    d. Normal finding in black patients

29. When would the nurse measure peripheral pulses?

    a. Any time the patient is admitted to the hospital

    b. When patients undergo vascular surgery

    c. When patients are more than 50 years of age

    d. When there is a history of cardiac problems

30. What is the cardinal sign of congestive heart failure?

    a. Murmurs

    b. Friction rub

    c. Gallops

    d. Snaps and clicks

31. What causes murmurs?

    a. Cardiac tamponade

    b. Congestive heart failure

    c. Turbulent blood flow through a valve

    d. Pericarditis

32. Major symptoms indicating alterations in the gastrointestinal system include:

    a. Heartburn

    b. Elevated white blood cell count

    c. Inability to discriminate taste

    d. Decreased creatine kinase level

33. A decreased fremitus may indicate:

    a. Atelectasis

    b. Pneumothorax

    c. Consolidation

    d. Chronic obstructive pulmonary disease

34. The patient is diagnosed with chronic bronchitis. The breath sounds will be described as:

    a. Rales

    b. Pleural friction rub

    c. Wheezing

    d. Rhonchi

35. Breath sounds that sound like fizzing seltzer, may be fine, medium, or coarse; wet or crackling sounds are called:

    a. Wheezing

    b. Pleural friction rub

    c. Rhonchi

    d. Rales

36. Periods of apnea followed by breath of increased depth are known as:

    a. Tachypnea

    b. Cheyne-Stokes breathing

c. Bitot breathing

d. Apnea

37. Breathing associated with severe brain stem damage that is completely chaotic and irregular is known as:

    a. Ataxic breathing

    b. Tachypnea

    c. Kussmaul breathing

    d. Cheyne-Stokes breathing

38. A decrease in the pH values of an arterial blood gas indicates:

    a. High altitude

    b. Lung disease

    c. Acidosis

    d. Polycythemia

39. Where would the nurse palpate the aorta?

    a. Epigastrium

    b. Apex

    c. Sternal notch

    d. Left midclavicular line

40. Normal bowel sounds should be heard in all four quadrants every:

    a. 5–20 seconds

    b. 60 seconds

    c. 2–5 minutes

    d. 10 minutes

41. Obese patients with musculoskeletal problems are at risk for:

    a. Calcium and protein deficiencies

    b. Decreased vitamin C intake

    c. Respiratory complications

    d. Weight-bearing problems

42. Inadequate exposure to sun predisposes the patient to:

    a. Excessive strains

    b. Bone and muscle tone loss

    c. Circulatory complications

    d. Cartilage degeneration

43. Sudden hypertension in a patient older than 50 years of age may indicate:

    a. Respiratory complications

    b. Cardiac dysrhythmia

    c. Cancer

    d. Renovascular disease

44. The inability to discriminate taste is associated with:

    a. Polycystic disease

    b. Prostatic disease

    c. Renal failure

    d. Hypertension

45. The diagnostic study used to visualize a joint is called:

    a. Gallium scan

    b. Arthrography

    c. Xeroradiography

    d. Indium imaging

46. The diagnostic test that determines the electrical potential generated in an individual muscle is called:

    a. Electromyography

    b. Magnetic resonance imaging

    c. Muscle biopsy

    d. Myelography

47. A decrease in urine output is known as:

    a. Dysuria

    b. Anuria

c. Hesitancy

d. Oliguria

48. The nursing diagnosis associated with a limited understanding of the injury or disease process and of the operative or invasive procedure is:

a. Knowledge deficit

b. Anticipatory anxiety

c. Ineffective individual coping

d. Fear

49. What will the patient use to alleviate anxiety and ensure a restful sleep?

a. Propanolol

b. Barbiturate

c. Atropine sulfate

d. Scopolamine hydrobromide

50. What are the precautions the nurse should take when administering chloral hydrate?

a. Give deep intramuscular injections

b. Maintain nothing-by-mouth status

c. Monitor heart rate

d. Monitor level of anxiety

✚ Answers

1. [c] Patient assessment

The nurse and the physician use assessment data. Assessment data are used by the nurse to diagnose actual or potential alterations in health that may affect the patient during the operative and invasive procedure period. (*page 17*)

2. [a] Establish the patient's risk of postprocedure complications

The physician uses the assessment data to diagnose acute or chronic medical conditions that may affect the performance of the procedure and to establish the patient's risk for postprocedure complications. (*page 17*)

3. [d] Establishes rapport

The nurse should establish contact with the patient by touching or shaking the patient's hand during the introduction. This helps to establish rapport and puts the patient at ease. Taking vital signs continues contact. (*page 17*)

4. [c] Introduce oneself

The nurse begins the assessment by introducing himself or herself to the patient and explaining the purpose of the assessment. Contact with the patient is established by touching or shaking the patient's hand during the introduction. (*page 17*)

5. [a] 23 months

If the patient is younger than 2 years of age, the age is recorded in months. (*page 18*)

6. [a] Proper calculation of medications

An accurate weight is critical for calculating medication dosage, especially for pediatric patients. Both weight and height help determine the patient's risk for adverse outcomes during the operative and invasive procedure period. (*page 18*)

7. [c] Renal failure

Possible postoperative complications for a patient with tachycardia include poor tissue perfusion, vascular collapse, cardiac arrhythmias, renal failure, and anesthetic complications. (*page 18*)

8. [b] 12–18 breaths/min

12–18 breaths/min is considered normal respiration. (*page 18*)

9. [d] Brain lesion

An abnormal finding of bradypnea, or less than 10 breaths/min, can be caused by a brain lesion or respiratory center depression. (*page 18*)

10. [d] Hemorrhage

An abnormal finding of hypertension can indicate anxiety, pain, or coronary artery disease. Possible postoperative complications include shock, stroke, hemorrhage, and myocardial infarction. (*page 18*)

11. [b] White blood cell count of 17,000 cells/mm

High leukocyte counts in patients undergoing elective procedures may be indicative of an unsuspected inflammatory process that could contraindicate the procedure. For example, an acute pneumonitis suggested by an elevated white blood cell count and confirmed by chest radiography necessitates cancellation of an elective procedure. (*page 19*)

12. [d] Hematocrit

If an anemic state is suspected, as in gastrointestinal bleeding, the hematocrit level aids in determining the need for blood replacement before the procedure. (*page 19*)

13. [b] Dehydration

The normal potassium range is 3.5–5 mEq/L. An increase would indicate dehydration or renal failure, and a decrease would indicate excessive use of diuretics, nausea, vomiting, hypotension, malnutrition, and cardiac arrhythmias. (*page 19*)

14. [b] Hyperventilation

Normal carbon dioxide range is 22–34 mEq/L. An increase would indicate chronic obstructive pulmonary disease, intestinal obstruction, or respiratory acidosis. A decrease would indicate hyperventilation, diabetic acidosis, or diarrhea. (*page 19*)

15. [a] Bone marrow depression

Extremely high white blood cell counts are rarely caused by infection alone and may suggest a leukemia condition. Unusually low counts might suggest bone marrow depression, which also contraindicates an elective procedure. (*page 19*)

16. [c] Dehydration

The normal blood urea nitrogen range is 5–15 mg/dL. An increase would indicate dehydration, renal failure, or excessive amounts of protein in the diet. A decrease would indicate overhydration, liver failure, or malnutrition. (*page 19*)

17. [a] Presence of syphilis

Serological blood determinations reflect heart and thyroid alterations as well as the presence of syphilis and infectious mononucleosis. (*page 20*)

18. [a] Infectious mononucleosis

Serological blood determinations reflect heart and thyroid alterations as well as the presence of syphilis and infectious mononucleosis. (*page 20*)

19. [d] Concentrated urine

Urine is normally pale yellow. Dark amber indicates concentrated urine; dark red or brown indicates blood in the urine or an increased urinary bilirubin level. Other color changes may result from diet or medications. (*page 20*)

20. [b] 12-Lead electrocardiogram (ECG)

A normal ECG does not eliminate the possibility of cardiac pathological changes, since the heart's muscle strength is not measured in this study. For patients with known cardiac disease, a 12-lead ECG is often undertaken to thoroughly evaluate electrical impulses in the heart. (*page 21*)

21. [c] Edematous tissue

Edematous tissue appears shiny, taut, and paler than uninvolved skin. (*page 25*)

22. [d] Cardiac insufficiency

Dependent or pitting edema may be caused by fluid and electrolyte imbalance and by venous and cardiac insufficiency. (*page 25*)

23. [a] Dorsum of the foot

Common sites of dependent or pitting edema are found on the dorsum of the foot and medial aspect of the ankle in ambulatory patients and on the buttocks, sacrum, and lower back of bedridden patients. (*page 25*)

24. [c] Endocrine imbalance

Endocrine imbalance may cause nonpitting edema, which is generalized but most easily seen over the tibia. (*page 25*)

25. [b] Increased serum carotene level

Yellow-orange skin color may be caused by increased total serum bilirubin, increased serum carotene level, and increased urochrome level. This can be a sign of liver disorders, pregnancy, thyroid deficiency, or diabetes. (*page 26*)

26. [a] Cardiomegaly

The patient should be assessed for cardiomegaly, which is present if the apex of the heart is percussed past the midclavicular line. (*page 27*)

27. [a] Jaundice

Diffuse yellow-brown discoloration of the nails indicates jaundice, peripheral lymphedema, bacterial fungal infection of the nail, psoriasis, and standing use of tobacco, nail polish, or dyes. (*page 27*)

28. [d] Normal finding in black patients

A vertical banding extending from the proximal nail fold distally is a normal finding in black patients. (*page 27*)

29. [b] When patients undergo vascular surgery

Peripheral pulses should be measured for patients undergoing angiography or cardiac or vascular surgery. Peripheral pulses include radial, ulnar, brachial, femoral, popliteal, dorsalis pedis, and posterior tibialis. (*page 28*)

30. [c] Gallops

Gallops are extra heart sounds that are best heard over the apex. They are the cardinal sign of congestive heart failure. (*page 28*)

31. [c] Turbulent blood flow through a valve

A murmur can be high or low pitched and is caused by turbulent blood flow through a valve as a result of congenital or acquired defects. (*page 28*)

32. [a] Heartburn

The major symptoms indicating alterations in the gastrointestinal system are belching, heartburn, bowel habit changes, weight loss, gastrointestinal bleeding, jaundice, and history of ulcers. Postprocedural complications include bleeding ulcers, liver failure, and intestinal obstruction. (*page 29*)

33. [b] Pneumothorax

A decreased fremitus may indicate pneumothorax or pleural effusion. Increased fremitus may indicate consolidation, secondary to atelectasis, or pneumonia. (*page 30*)

34. [d] Rhonchi

Rhonchi are characterized as bubbling or rumbling sounds and are significant for chronic bronchitis or any disorder with retained pulmonary secretions. (*page 30*)

35. [d] Rales

Rales sound like fizzing seltzer; they may be fine, medium, or coarse, and wet or crackling. Rales are indicative of pulmonary edema (wet) or pulmonary fibrosis (dry). (*page 30*)

36. [b] Cheyne-Stokes breathing

Periods of apnea followed by breath of increased depth is known as Cheyne-Stokes breathing. This breathing can be caused by increased intracranial pressure, severe congestive heart failure, renal failure, meningitis, drug overdose, or cerebral anoxia. (*page 31*)

37. [a] Ataxic breathing

Breathing associated with severe brain stem damage that is completely chaotic and irregular is known as ataxic breathing. (*page 31*)

38. [c] Acidosis

Normal range of pH is 7.35–7.45. An increase is indicative of alkalosis; a decrease is indicative of acidosis. (*page 31*)

39. [a] Epigastrium

The aorta is often palpable at the epigastrium slightly left of the midline. The aorta feels like a long, thin, consistent, pulsatile mass. An enlarged area may indicate an aneurysm. (*page 31*)

40. [a] 5–20 seconds

Normal bowel sounds should be heard in all four quadrants every 5–20 seconds. (*page 32*)

41. [c] Respiratory complications

Obese patients with musculoskeletal problems are at risk for respiratory and circulatory complications. Obesity also places excessive strain and stress on joints and bones, which may lead to fractures and cartilage degeneration. (*page 33*)

42. [b] Bone and muscle tone loss

One must determine whether the patient is regularly exposed to sunlight. Inadequate exposure predisposes the patient to bone and muscle loss. (*page 33*)

43. [d] Renovascular disease

Some urinary tract disorders are related to the age or gender of the patient. For example, sudden hypertension in a patient more than 50 years of age may indicate the presence of renovascular disease. (*page 33*)

44. [c] Renal failure

Symptoms such as changes in appetite and taste acuity and an inability to discriminate tastes are associated with the accumulation of nitrogenous waste products from renal disease. (*page 33*)

45. [b] Arthrography

Arthrography visualizes a joint after injection of a contrast medium (air or solution) to enhance visualization. (*page 35*)

46. [a] Electromyography

Electromyography is used to determine the electrical potential generated in an individual muscle. Usually accompanied by nerve conduction studies, it is helpful in the diagnosis of neuromuscular, lower motor neuron, and peripheral nerve disorder. (*page 35*)

47. [d] Oliguria

Oliguria is a decrease in urine output, specifically an ouput of 100–400 mL/24 hours. (*page 36*)

48. [a] Knowledge deficit

Defining characteristics for knowledge deficit include limited understanding of the injury or disease process and of the operative or invasive procedure, poor performance of a required skill, and inaccurate or inappropriate responses to questions about the operative or invasive procedure. (*page 38*)

49. [b] Barbiturate

To alleviate patient anxiety and to ensure a restful sleep, a barbiturate or sleeping pill may be prescribed the night before the procedure for inpatients. One to 2 hours before the procedure, or sometimes immediately before the procedure, medications may be given to the patient to alleviate anxiety. (*page 40*)

50. [d] Monitor level of anxiety

Cloral hydrate is a sedative that is given 0.5–1 g by mouth. The nurse should monitor the respiratory status and level of anxiety, and encourage verbalization and relaxation. (*page 41*)

CHAPTER **3**

Transferring the Patient

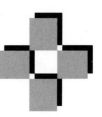

Transferring the patient describes the activities done by the nurse or other members of the operative and invasive procedure nursing team to move the patient to and from the operative and invasive procedure suite without tissue injury, altered body temperature, ineffective breathing patterns, altered tissue perfusion, discomfort, or pain. The questions for this chapter will help the reader assess his or her knowledge about

• Identifying the patient's risk for adverse outcomes related to transfer activities
• Transferring the patient to the operative and invasive procedure suite holding area
• Admitting the patient to the operative and invasive procedure suite holding area
• Transferring the patient from the holding area to the procedure room
• Transferring the patient from the procedure room to the postanesthesia care unit
• Transferring the patient from the operative and invasive procedure suite to the nursing unit after local anesthesia
• Transferring the patient with special needs
• Documentation and communication procedures

The reference used for this chapter is Phippen, M. L., & Wells, M. P. (1999). *Patient care during operative and invasive procedures.* Philadelphia: W. B. Saunders, pp. 45–53.

✚ Questions

1. The pregnant patient is at risk for altered tissue perfusion while being transferred to the operative and invasive procedure

suite. Risk factors associated with this nursing diagnosis are:

a. Anxiety and improper positioning during transfer

b. Supine position and third trimester of pregnancy

c. Prone position and first trimester of pregnancy

d. Left lateral position and third trimester of pregnancy

2. Select the condition below that best describes a risk factor for the diagnosis *Risk for Injury related to transfer to and from the operative and invasive procedure suite.*

a. Cold environment

b. Altered metabolic rate

c. Neuromuscular impairment

d. Anxiety

3. After an upper endoscopy procedure in the gastrointestional laboratory, the nurse prepares for transfer of the patient to the outpatient care unit. The patient, who weighs 350 lb and is 5 feet 6 inches tall, received intravenous conscious sedation during the procedure. Based on these data, the most appropriate nursing diagnosis is:

a. Risk for Discomfort during transfer to the outpatient care unit

b. Risk for Altered Body Temperature during transfer to the outpatient care unit

c. Risk for Injury during transfer to the outpatient care unit

Mohawk Valley Community College Library

d. Risk for Ineffective Breathing Pattern during transfer to the outpatient care unit

4. Select the statement that does not describe an acceptable measurement criterion for the outcome standard *Transfer activities implemented during the operative and invasive procedure period do not compromise or cause injury to the patient.*

a. The patient is free from evidence of positional injury.

b. The patient is free from evidence of tissue injury.

c. The patient is free from evidence of altered tissue perfusion.

d. The patient is free from evidence of altered body temperature.

5. What is the first thing the nursing assistant should do after receiving the patient transfer assignment?

a. Obtain a transportation vehicle and immediately depart for the patient care unit

b. Obtain a transportation vehicle and clean it before departing the operative and invasive procedure suite

c. Confer with the charge nurse of the operative and invasive procedure suite concerning transportation equipment requirements and planned patient care activities during the transfer

d. Call the patient care unit and speak to the charge nurse to determine patient care requirements during the transfer period

6. Family members usually play an important role in decreasing the patient's anxiety about the operative or invasive procedure. Family members should:

a. Remain in the patient's room

b. Accompany the patient to the operative and invasive procedure suite

c. Go immediately to the waiting room

d. Help guide the gurney through the hallway

7. Patient identification is important to:

a. Decrease patient anxiety

b. Ensure that the correct physician's name is on chart

c. Be sure that the patient knows what is really going to be done to him or her

d. Ensure that the correct patient is transported

8. After arriving in the patient's room, the transporter should:

a. Allow the unit nurse to tell the patient it is time to leave the nursing unit

b. Tell the patient it is time for the procedure

c. Instruct family members to help the patient to the gurney

d. Assist the patient to the toilet to void one last time

9. The first thing a transporter should do when he or she reaches the holding area with a patient is:

a. Tell the charge nurse the patient has arrived

b. Give the patient a warm blanket

c. Lock the wheels on the gurney

d. Document time of arrival on the patient chart

10. After arriving on the unit, the transporter will first:

a. Introduce himself or herself to patient

b. Ask whether the patient is ready to depart for the operative and invasive procedure suite

c. Report to the patient's nurse

d. Request that unit personnel assist with moving the patient to the gurney

11. The mother of an 11-year-old female patient signed the consent for an invasive procedure 2 days before the procedure. By prior arrangement, the mother is not present when the patient is taken to the operative and invasive procedure suite. Who should identify the patient?

    a. The unit nurse should identify the patient.

    b. The physician should identify the patient.

    c. The wrist band should be used to identify the patient.

    d. The patient is old enough to identify herself.

12. To prevent a patient from experiencing motion sickness, the transporter will:

    a. Push the patient feet first

    b. Push the patient head first

    c. Pull the patient so he or she has someone to look at

    d. Ask for help to transport the patient

13. Bill Higgins, a 23-year-old single man, was brought into the emergency department in a coma. He was accompanied by his mother. Mr. Higgins will be identified by:

    a. Physician

    b. Ambulance driver

    c. Police officer

    d. Family member

14. The gurney should be pulled out of the elevator by the transporter to allow:

    a. Transporter to clear the hallway

    b. Transporter to hold the door open

    c. Patient to see a familiar face

    d. Patient to have a degree of privacy from visitors

15. The transporter will review the patient consent form to be sure it is:

    a. On the cart

    b. Dated and witnessed by family members

    c. Typed and signed by the patient

    d. Signed and witnessed according to hospital policy and procedure

16. Who should go to the patient's room with the transporter?

    a. Another transporter

    b. Family members

    c. Unit nursing personnel

    d. Circulating nurse

17. After the transporter has greeted the patient, he or she should:

    a. Introduce himself or herself

    b. Greet the patient by her or his full name

    c. Ask what type of procedure the patient is undergoing

    d. Read the patient's wristband

18. If facility protocols have not been followed in obtaining an informed signed consent (barring emergency situations), what should be done?

    a. The anesthesia provider should be notified.

    b. The patient should be asked why protocol was not followed.

    c. The family should be notified.

    d. The procedure should be postponed until a valid consent form is obtained.

19. If a preprocedure assessment has not been done, the holding area nurse will:

    a. Tell the circulating nurse that the assessment needs to be done

b. Report this information to the physician

c. Do an assessment

d. Ask the unit nurse to come to the holding area to do an assessment

20. If blood has been ordered but is not in the operative-invasive procedure suite refrigerator, the holding area nurse should:

a. Draw blood from patient and send to laboratory for typing

b. Call the laboratory to be sure the order was received

c. Ask the patient if the laboratory drew blood the night before

d. Send family members to laboratory to donate blood

21. The nurse validated nothing-by-mouth (NPO) status by:

a. Checking the chart

b. Asking the transporter

c. Calling the unit nurse

d. Asking the patient

22. Which team member remains at the patient's head while the mobile patient is transferred to the procedure bed from the gurney?

a. Circulating nurse

b. Physician

c. Anesthesia provider

d. No one is necessary at the head since the patient is not asleep

23. Why would the circulator announce that the patient is entering the operative and invasive procedure suite?

a. To alert personnel to reduce the noise level

b. To include the patient in current conversation

c. To stop all conversation

d. To have all personnel except the circulator vacate the room

24. How is the patient's privacy maintained during transfer to procedure bed?

a. Ask all nonessential personnel to leave the room

b. Keep cover sheet in place

c. Allow the patient to keep pajamas on

d. Keep all blankets in place until transfer is made

25. What is the minimum amount of personnel needed for safe transfer of an immobile patient?

a. Two

b. Six

c. Four

d. Three

26. To ensure that the safety strap is secured properly, the circulating nurse will:

a. Check the popliteal pulse

b. Be able to place one hand between the strap and the patient's thighs

c. Place a blanket between the strap and the patient's legs

d. Be able to place one fist between strap and the patient's legs

27. When moving a patient, the side lifter's upper torso should be:

a. Bent slightly forward

b. Turned slightly to the left

c. Bent slightly back for support

d. Straight

28. What patient may respond more combat-
    ively during the excitement phase of
    the anesthesia?

    a. Football player

    b. Physician

    c. Piano player

    d. Waitperson

29. The mobile patient is instructed to move
    from his or her bed to gurney:

    a. Buttocks first, shoulders second, feet
       last

    b. Shoulders first, buttocks second, feet
       last

    c. Feet first, buttocks second, shoulders
       last

    d. Patient never moves by himself or
       herself

30. Safety strap is placed:

    a. 2 inches below the knees

    b. Across the waist

    c. 2 inches above the knees

    d. Anywhere below the waist

31. During the bed-tilt technique, the gur-
    ney is:

    a. Tight against the procedure bed

    b. Slightly away from the procedure bed

    c. Unlocked to facilitate transfer

    d. It does not matter

32. Which member of the nursing team ac-
    companies the patient to the postanes-
    thesia care unit?

    a. Orderly

    b. Surgical technologist

    c. Nurse

    d. Anesthesia provider

33. What is the most dangerous time of
    transfer for the elective operative pa-
    tient?

    a. Transfer from the nursing unit to the
       operative-invasive procedure suite

    b. Transfer from the operative and
       invasive procedure suite to the
       postanesthesia care unit

    c. Transfer from the holding area to the
       operative and invasive procedure suite

    d. Transfer from the postanesthesia care
       unit to the nursing unit

34. The bed-tilt transfer creates a slope be-
    tween the bed and the gurney. This gradi-
    ent facilitates transfer with:

    a. Need for fewer personnel

    b. Mobile patients

    c. Small children

    d. Minimal stress on lifters and the
       patient

35. The report the nurse gives the postanes-
    thesia care unit nurse should include:

    a. Type of procedure performed and
       anesthesia used

    b. Type of intravenous solution hung and
       family member whereabouts

    c. Patient condition, nursing care
       provided during the procedure, and
       dressing location

    d. Type of procedure and name of surgeon

36. If transfer of a local patient to the nursing
    unit is delayed, the patient will:

    a. Be sent to floor and the unit nursing
       manager will deal with the crisis

    b. Be discharged from postanesthesia
       care unit to home

    c. Remain in the operative and invasive
       procedure suite until a hospital unit
       can accommodate the patient

    d. Be transported to appropriate holding
       area until the nursing unit is ready

37. Before a patient who has received a local anesthetic is transferred to the nursing unit:

   a. The patient should be assessed to determine whether a nurse should accompany him or her to the unit

   b. Intravenous fluids should be discontinued

   c. The dressing should be checked and intravenous fluids should be discontinued

   d. The anesthesia provider should write an order allowing the patient to return directly to the nursing care unit

38. Transferring a patient with a lower extremity fracture that has been stabilized with an external device to the operative and invasive procedure suite is different from transferring an elderly patient because:

   a. The patient with a traction device is transferred in his or her bed

   b. The patient with a traction device is allowed to have family members in the holding area

   c. The surgeon accompanies the patient with traction

   d. The nurse must accompany the patient with traction

39. If a patient from the intensive care unit requires respiratory assistance, he or she should be accompanied by a nurse from the operative and invasive procedure suite or by an intensive care unit nurse and:

   a. Physician

   b. Orderlies to transport

   c. Respiratory therapist or anesthesia provider

   d. Postanesthesia care nurse

40. Toddlers who are difficult to restrain should be transported in a:

   a. Crib

   b. Wheelchair

   c. Crib with a bubble top

   d. Bed with side rails up

41. A neonate patient is not transferred to the operative and invasive procedure suite until:

   a. The parents have taken a tour of the operative and invasive procedure suite

   b. The procedure room has been warmed and prepared for the procedure

   c. The neonate can maintain his or her own body temperature at 36.8°C (98.2°F)

   d. The surgeon is ready to make the incision

42. The transporter must document:

   a. Method of transfer, time of arrival in and departure from the operative and invasive procedure suite, and name of transporter

   b. Method of transfer, who accompanied patient to the operative and invasive procedure suite, and name of unit nurse assigned to patient

   c. Name of transporter, time of arrival to the operative and invasive procedure suite, and name of physician

   d. Name of physician, circulating nurse accepting the patient, and type of procedure to be performed

✚ Answers

1. [b] Supine position and third trimester of pregnancy

   Risk factors associated with this nursing diagnosis are supine position and third trimester of pregnancy. (*page 47*)

2. [c] Neuromuscular impairment

   Risk factors for the diagnosis *Risk for Injury related to transfer to and from the operative and invasive procedure suite* include neuromuscular impairment, musculoskeletal impairment, vascular impairment, cognitive impairment, sensory/perceptual impairment (vision, hearing), speech impairment, safety violations by the transporter, equipment malfunction, and extraneous objects such as hanging intravenous bags and drainage devices. (*page 47*)

3. [d] Risk for Ineffective Breathing Pattern during transfer to the outpatient care unit

Risk factors for the diagnosis of *Risk for Ineffective Breathing Pattern during transfer to the outpatient care unit* include obesity, preprocedure sedation, neuromuscular impairment, musculoskeletal impairment, perceptual or cognitive impairment, anxiety, pain, improper position of the patient during transfer, and third trimester of pregnancy. (*page 47*)

4. [a] The patient is free from evidence of positional injury.

Acceptable measurement criteria for the outcome standard *Transfer activities implemented during the operative and invasive procedure period do not compromise or cause injury to the patient:* patient will be free from evidence of tissue injury, altered body temperature, ineffective breathing pattern, altered tissue perfusion, and discomfort and pain. (*page 46*)

5. [c] Confer with the charge nurse of the operative and invasive procedure suite concerning transportation equipment requirements and planned patient care activities during the transfer

After the patient transfer assignment has been received, one must confer with the nurse or review the nursing care plan to check for orders concerning transportation equipment requirements and planned patient care activities during the transfer. (*page 45*)

6. [b] Accompany the patient to the operative and invasive procedure suite

If present, family members or significant others should accompany the patient to the operative and invasive procedure suite. This may help minimize the patient's anxiety about the impending procedure. (*page 46*)

7. [d] Ensure that the correct patient is transported

Identification of the patient ensures that the correct patient is transported to the operative and invasive procedure suite at the appropriate time with all necessary paperwork completed and in the chart. (*page 46*)

8. [a] Allow the unit nurse to tell the patient it is time to leave the nursing unit

Unit nursing personnel should accompany the transporter to the patient's room or cubicle to perform the preliminary identification of the patient and assist with the transfer process. After arriving in the patient's room, the unit nurse tells the patient that it is time to depart for the operative and invasive procedure suite. (*page 46*)

9. [c] Lock the wheels on the gurney

When in the holding area, the wheels of the gurney should be locked and the holding area nurse and suite patient care coordinator told that the patient has arrived. (*page 48*)

10. [c] Report to the patient's nurse

After arriving on the nursing unit, one should report to the patient's nurse, ask whether the patient is ready to depart for the operative and invasive procedure suite, and request that unit personnel assist with moving the patient to the gurney. (*page 46*)

11. [a] The unit nurse should identify the patient.

If a parent or legal guardian is unavailable, rely on the unit nursing staff to identify the patient. This does not negate the need to check the transfer slip against the patient's identification bracelet and chart. (*page 46*)

12. [a] Push the patient feet first.

Pushing the patient feet first allows the patient to see where he or she is going. Also, some patients may experience motion sickness if moved backward. (*page 47*)

13. [d] Family member

If a family member or a significant other is present, the nurse should ask him or her to identify the comatose patient. (*page 46*)

14. [b] Transporter to hold the door open

When the gurney is being pulled out of the elevator, the elevator doors should be held back to prevent inadvertent closure on the gurney. (*page 46*)

15. [d] Signed and witnessed according to hospital policy and procedure

Before entering the patient's room or cubicle, one must review the patient's chart and check the procedure consent form for patient and witness signatures according to the policy of the healthcare facility. (*page 46*)

16. [c] Unit nursing personnel

Unit nursing personnel should accompany the transporter to the patient's room to perform the preliminary identification of the patient and to assist with the transfer process. (*page 46*)

17. [b] Greet the patient by her or his full name

After entering the patient's room or cubicle, one should greet the patient by her or his full name. Next, the transporter identifies himself or herself and then asks the patient to say his or her name and what procedure she or he is having done. (*page 46*)

18. [d] The procedure should be postponed until a valid consent form is obtained.

If facility protocols have not been followed in obtaining an informed signed consent (barring emergency situations), a valid consent must be obtained before the procedure is begun. Patients with a cognitive impairment or with altered sensorium secondary to preprocedure medication should not sign a consent form. When the patient is no longer affected by the medication, the physician counsels the patient again, and a new consent form is signed and witnessed according to facility policy. (*page 48*)

19. [c] Do an assessment

If an assessment has not been done, the holding area nurse should perform an assessment. After the assessment, the holding area nurse gives the assessment data to the nurse assigned to provide patient care during the procedure. (*page 48*)

20. [b] Call the laboratory to be sure the order was received

If blood has been ordered, one should check with the patient care coordinator to ensure that the blood is available. If the blood is not available, one must call the laboratory to ensure that the order has been received and to check blood availability. (*page 48*)

21. [d] Asking the patient

The nurse validates NPO status by asking the patient the last time he or she had something to eat or drink. (*page 48*)

22. [d] No one is necessary at the head since the patient is not asleep

During the transfer of a mobile patient, the circulating nurse stands next to the gurney. The anesthesia provider or assistive person stands on the opposite side of the bed to protect the patient from falling off the bed during transfer. (*page 48*)

23. [a] To alert personnel to reduce the noise level

On entering the procedure room, the circulator announces to team members that the patient is entering the room. This alerts the staff in the room that noise must be kept to a minimum. (*page 48*)

24. [b] Keep cover sheet in place

The patient's privacy is protected by keeping the cover sheet in place during the transfer. (*page 49*)

25. [c] Four

Depending on the patient's size, at least four people should move an immobile patient. (*page 49*)

26. [b] Be able to place one hand between the strap and the patient's thighs

The strap is checked for excessive tautness or looseness by placing one hand between the patient's thighs and the strap. (*page 49*)

27. [d] Straight

During the transfer of a patient, the side lifter maintains his or her upper torso in a straight and upright position. (*page 49*)

28. [a] Football player

Patients employed in physically demanding occupations or aggressive hobbies sometimes respond more combatively during the excitement phase of anesthesia than do other patients. (*page 49*)

29. [a] Buttocks first, shoulders second, feet last

The circulating nurse asks the mobile patient to move to the bed, moving buttocks first, shoulders second, and feet last. (*page 49*)

30. [c] 2 inches above the knees

The circulating nurse places a safety strap across the patient's thighs, approximately 2 inches (5 cm) above the knees. (*page 49*)

31. [b] Slightly away from the procedure bed

During the bed-tilt technique, the circulator moves the recovery bed slightly away from the bed to allow the anesthesia provider to operate the lever and thus tilt the bed. (*page 49*)

32. [c] Nurse

The patient may not be fully recovered from the effects of the anesthetic agents and thus is dependent on the procedure team members for basic support such as airway management. Therefore, the nurse must implement the patient care activities with the anesthesia provider. (*page 49*)

33. [b] Transfer from the operative and invasive procedure suite to the postanesthesia care unit

Transfer from the procedure room to the postanesthesia care unit is potentially the most dangerous time for the patient during the transfer process. The patient may not be fully recovered from the effects of the anesthetic agents and thus is dependent on the procedure team members for basic support such as airway management. (*page 49*)

34. [d] Minimal stress on lifters and the patient

The gradient facilitates patient transfer with minimal stress on the lifters and the patient. (*page 50, Fig. 4.2*)

35. [c] Patient condition, nursing care provided during the procedure, and dressing location

At a minimum, the report given by the nurse to the postanesthesia care unit nurse should include the patient's condition, nursing care provided during the procedure, and the location of dressing and drainage devices. (*page 51*)

36. [d] Be transported to appropriate holding area until the nursing unit is ready

If transport to the nursing unit is delayed, the patient should be taken to the holding area to await transfer back to the nursing unit. (*page 52*)

37. [a] The patient should be assessed to determine whether a nurse should accompany him or her to the unit

The local patient should be assessed before transfer to the unit to determine whether a nurse should accompany him or her to the unit. (*page 52*)

38. [a] The patient with a traction device is transferred in his or her bed

Before transporting the patient with an orthopedic injury, the nurse must assess the patient to determine the extent of injury, the traction or immobilization devices in use, and the appropriate vehicle for transfer. In general, a patient with extensive injuries and multiple skeletal support devices is transported to the operative and invasive procedure suite in an orthopedic bed. (*page 52*)

39. [c] Respiratory therapist or anesthesia provider

An operative and invasive procedure nurse or intensive care nurse should accompany all patients from the intensive care unit. If a critically ill patient requires respiratory assistance, an anesthesia provider or a respiratory therapist should accompany him or her. (*page 52*)

40. [c] Crib with a bubble top

Toddlers and other children who are noncooperative, such as those who refuse to remain lying and who are secured with a safety strap, should be transported in a crib with a bubble top and the side rails up. (*page 52*)

41. [b] The procedure room has been warmed and prepared for the procedure

Like intensive care patients, infants should be taken directly to the procedure room, unless the holding area is equipped and staffed to provide. The infant is not transferred until the procedure room is warmed and prepared for the procedure. (*page 52*)

42. [a] Method of transfer, time of arrival in and departure from the operative and invasive procedure suite, and name of transporter

The transporter documents transfer activities according to hospital policy and procedure. At a minimum, documentation by the transporter must include the method of transfer, the time of arrival in and departure from the operative and invasive procedure suite, and the identity of the person who transported the patient. (*page 53*)

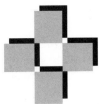

CHAPTER 4

Assisting the
Anesthesia Provider

The practice of anesthesia is an integral part of patient care not only in hospital-based operating rooms but also in surgery centers, physician's offices, and other outpatient facilities. Therefore, assisting the anesthesia provider is an important role of the nurse providing care to the patient undergoing an operative and invasive procedure that requires anesthesia. The questions for this chapter will help the reader assess his or her knowledge about

• Preprocedure assessment
• Preinduction
• Induction of, maintenance of, and emergence from anesthesia
• Special situations

The reference used for this chapter is Phippen, M. L., & Wells, M. P. (1999). *Patient care during operative and invasive procedure.* Philadelphia: W. B. Saunders, pp. 54–60.

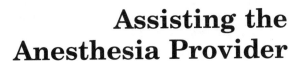

Questions

1. The responsibility of ensuring that appropriate assistance is given to meet the anesthetic needs of the patient rests with:

   a. Anesthesiologist

   b. Surgeon

   c. Circulating nurse

   d. Scrub nurse

2. The first step toward ensuring patient readiness for an operative or invasive procedure is:

   a. Preprocedure assessment by both the anesthesia care provider and perioperative nurse

   b. Administration of a sedative to relax the patient

   c. Positioning the patient for comfort

   d. Having all noise in the procedure suite kept to a minimum

3. When does the anesthesia assessment of inpatients usually take place?

   a. The day of the procedure

   b. The night before the procedure

   c. At the time the procedure is scheduled

   d. At the time the decision is made to have a procedure

4. According to the American Society of Anesthesiology, the status of a patient with no organic, physiological, biochemical, or psychiatric disturbances would be classified as:

   a. Class 4

   b. Class 3

   c. Class 2

   d. Class 1

5. During Mrs. Thomas's anesthesia assessment, it was determined that her blood pressure was 172/94. The American Society of Anesthesiology physical status classification for Mrs. Thomas would be:

   a. Class 1

   b. Class 2

   c. Class 3

   d. Class 4

6. According to the American Society of Anesthesiology classification system, which patient would be classified as a class 3?

   a. A patient with no physiological disturbances

   b. A patient with hypertension

   c. A patient with hypertension and a history of myocardial infarction

   d. A patient with little chance of survival

7. Mr. Morgan has been diagnosed with a ruptured abdominal aneurysm. The anesthesia care provider assesses him and determines his physical status classification to be:

   a. Class 2

   b. Class 3

   c. Class 4

   d. Class 5

8. If an unusual finding is discovered during the nursing preoperative assessment, the nurse should:

   a. Document it in the nursing notes

   b. Discuss the finding with the patient's family or significant other for clarification

   c. Report the findings to the anesthesia care provider

   d. Share the findings with the postanesthesia care unit

9. When should the patient be brought to the operative or invasive procedure suite?

   a. When the physician asks the nurse to bring the patient into the suite

   b. When the suite is ready

   c. Immediately after the preoperative assessment

   d. As soon as possible

10. Why is soft music played in the operative or invasive procedure suite?

    a. Decreases patient anxiety

    b. Masks the noise of the suction equipment

    c. Physician preference

    d. Music should not be played

11. What are the two components needed to provide successful anesthesia for patients requiring regional anesthesia?

    a. Nonimpaired drug metabolism and prevention of cross-contamination

    b. Negative nitrogen balance and decreased drug metabolism

    c. Thermoregulation and pain control

    d. Adequate amnesia and analgesia

12. Why are medications from the benzodiazepine family used to produce amnesia?

    a. Decreases chance of nausea after the procedure

    b. Decreases cardiovascular depression

    c. Decreases pain tolerance

    d. Increases nitrogen levels

13. The major side effect of opioids is:

    a. Respiratory depression

    b. Erythema

    c. Insomnia

    d. Tachycardia

14. The most commonly used opioid is:

    a. Morphine

    b. Diazepam

    c. Fentanyl

    d. Midazolam

15. A complication of hypothermia is:

    a. Postprocedure positive nitrogen balance

    b. Decreased pain intolerance

c. Potential for wound evisceration

d. Decreased drug metabolism

16. What position will the patient be placed in to receive a regional block?

a. Prone

b. Sitting

c. Supine

d. Semi-Fowler's

17. How long will the effects of a spinal anesthetic last?

a. 10–30 minutes

b. 30 minutes to 3 hours

c. 3–5 hours

d. 8–10 hours

18. Mrs. Burns is being admitted to the labor and delivery unit. The anesthesia choice for her would be:

a. Spinal anesthesia

b. Epidural block

c. Bier block

d. General anesthesia

19. The most common concern with induction of a spinal anesthesia is:

a. Hypotension

b. Pain relief

c. Vasoconstriction

d. Amnesia

20. What could happen if, during the invasive procedure, the tourniquet used for a Bier block malfunctions?

a. Patient will experience pain during the procedure.

b. Patient will be overmedicated.

c. Patient will experience severe nausea during the procedure.

d. Patient will experience immediate headache.

21. What drug will the nurse prepare in the event of toxic blood levels after the tourniquet is released?

a. Diazepam

b. Propofol

c. Morphine

d. Fentanyl

22. The stage of anesthesia induction that is known as the excitement phase is:

a. Stage 4

b. Stage 3

c. Stage 2

d. Stage 1

23. At what stage will paralysis of the diaphragm be present?

a. Stage 1

b. Stage 2

c. Stage 3

d. Stage 4

24. Where should the circulating nurse be during induction of general anesthesia?

a. At the patient's head

b. At the back table, assisting the scrub nurse with counting instrumentation

c. At the scrub sink, observing the scrub technique of new medical residents

d. At the patient's side, prepared to assist the anesthesia care provider

25. To effectively close off the esophagus and allow better visualization of the vocal cords for intubation, the circulating nurse will:

a. Administer oxygen through a nasal cannula

b. Position the patient in the semi-Fowler's position

c. Apply cricoid pressure

d. Deflate the balloon on the endotracheal tube

26. A common problem associated with inhalation agents is:

a. Irritation of the larynx

b. Swelling of the tissue around the trachea

c. Deviation of the trachea

d. Respiratory failure

27. If ketamine is used as the anesthetic agent, before the patient emergence from anesthesia, the circulating nurse will:

a. Dim the lights

b. Notify the postanesthesia care unit

c. Administer morphine

d. Secure extra help for transporting the patient

28. A cause of postoperative agitation may be:

a. Toxic medication levels

b. Hypoxia

c. Nitrogen depletion

d. Hyperthermia

29. Who has the responsibility to transfuse the patient during the operative or invasive procedure?

a. Circulating nurse

b. Scrub person

c. Surgeon

d. Anesthesia provider

30. What is the induction of choice for an emergency operative or invasive procedure?

a. Rapid sequence induction

b. Spinal anesthesia

c. Inhalation sequence

d. Dissociative anesthesia

31. What is the danger of rapid sequence induction of general anesthesia in an emergency situation?

a. Drug toxicity

b. Poor positioning after induction

c. Potential for hypothermia

d. Vomiting of stomach contents

32. A hypermetabolic state that results in increased carbon dioxide production, oxygen consumption, and muscle membrane destruction is known as:

a. Cushingoid syndrome

b. Malignant hyperthermia

c. Diabetic insufficiency

d. Paget disease

33. What is the triggering agent for malignant hyperthermia?

a. Morphine

b. Atropine

c. Succinylcholine

d. Dantrolene

34. What is the drug for treatment of malignant hyperthermia?

a. Succinylcholine

b. Valium

c. Diazepam

d. Dantrolene

35. The first step in the treatment of malignant hyperthermia is:

a. Surgeon request to close as quickly as possible

b. Request for malignant hyperthermia kit

c. Discontinuation of anesthesia

d. Hyperventilation with 100% oxygen

Answers

1. [c] Circulating nurse

Many care providers may be involved with helping the anesthesia provider, such as anesthesia technicians, licensed practical nurses, and unlicensed assistive personnel. It is the responsibility of the circulating nurse to ensure that appropriate assistance is given to meet the anesthetic needs of the patient. (*page 54*)

2. [a] Preprocedure assessment by both the anesthesia care provider and perioperative nurse

Preoperative assessment is the first step toward ensuring patient readiness for an operative or invasive procedure from both the nursing and anesthesia perspectives. The assessment is necessary and helpful in determining the patient's history and present physical, mental, and emotional status. (*page 54*)

3. [b] The night before the procedure

A preprocedure assessment is performed by a member of the anesthesia team before the patient's arrival in the operative and invasive procedure holding area. This assessment is done on an outpatient basis for patients who arrive the day of the procedure. The anesthesia assessment of inpatients usually takes place the night before the procedure. (*page 54*)

4. [d] Class 1

Class 1: A patient with no organic, physiological, biochemical, or psychological disturbances. (*page 54*)

5. [b] Class 2

Class 2: Mild to moderate systemic disturbances caused by a condition to be treated surgically or by a pathophysiological process, such as hypertension or diabetes. (*page 54*)

6. [c] A patient with hypertension and a history of myocardial infarction

Class 3: Severe systemic diseases with more than one system involved, such as hypertension, cardiac disease, and pulmonary problems. (*page 54*)

7. [d] Class 5

Class 5: A patient who has little chance of survival. The operative procedure may be a resuscitative measure with little anesthesia, such as a ruptured abdominal aneurysm or major cerebral trauma with rapidly increasing intracranial pressure. (*page 55*)

8. [c] Report the findings to the anesthesia care provider

Nursing assessment tools and the documentation should be complete and concise. Any unusual findings should be reported to the anesthetist. (*page 55*)

9. [b] When the suite is ready

The patient should never be brought to the operative and invasive procedure suite until it is absolutely ready. Scurrying about once the patient is brought into the procedure room only heightens the patient's fears. (*page 55*)

10. [a] Decreases patient anxiety

Many procedure rooms have soft music playing in the background, which has a tendency to decrease anxiety and soothe the patient. It is of the utmost importance to keep the noise and activity levels to a minimum. (*page 55*)

11. [d] Adequate amnesia and analgesia

There are two components that are needed to provide successful anesthesia for patients who require monitored sedation or regional anesthesia. Goals for the anesthesia care provider in this situation are safe and adequate amnesia and analgesia during the procedure. (*page 55*)

12. [b] Decreases cardiovascular depression

Medications from the benzodiazepine family are used because they produce amnesia and are associated with less cardiovascular and respiratory depression. The commonly used benzodiazepines are diazepam, lorazepam, and midazolam. (*page 55*)

13. [a] Respiratory depression

Opioids decrease the sensation of pain as well as alter the patient's response to pain. Although the perception or sensation of pain may be altered, the other sensory responses remain functional. The major side effects of opioids are respiratory depression, nausea, and vomiting. (*page 55*)

14. [c] Fentanyl

The most commonly used opioid is fentanyl, which is more potent than morphine. (*page 55*)

15. [d] Decreased drug metabolism

Prevention of hypothermia is important because complications arising from hypothermia include decreased drug metabolism, impaired coagulation, increased local anesthetic toxicity, impaired response to wound infections, thermal discomfort, postprocedural negative nitrogen balance, and shivering. (*page 56*)

16. [b] Sitting

The patient who is to receive a regional block such as a spinal or epidural block as an adjunct to sedation may be placed in either a side-lying position or a sitting position. (*page 56*)

17. [b] 30 minutes to 3 hours

Spinal anesthesia involves injecting a local anesthetic into the subarachnoid space. The medication is quickly absorbed in the nerve fibers, and a loss of sensation and controlled movement occurs. This type of block lasts from 30 minutes to 3 hours. (*page 56*)

18. [b] Epidural block

The patient receiving an epidural block may not lose as much motor function as he or she would with a spinal block. There is a lower incidence of headache with an epidural block, and an epidural block may be placed before general anesthesia and is then used to control postoperative pain. An epidural anesthetic is also used frequently for patients in labor and delivery. (*page 56*)

19. [a] Hypotension

The most common concern with induction of spinal anesthesia (less so with an epidural block) is hypotension. This is caused by peripheral vasodilatation, which in turn causes hypovolemia and a fall in blood pressure. (*page 56*)

20. [b] Patient will be overmedicated.

The bier block consists of using a double tourniquet and administering the anesthetic agent intravenously. If the tourniquet malfunctions or is applied improperly, a potentially dangerous dose of medication could enter the systemic circulation. (*page 56*)

21. [a] Diazepam

If toxic blood levels are reached, a seizure may occur. The nurse must be prepared to use all seizure precautions, including assisting the anesthetist with the administration of both oxygen and a sedative, such as diazepam. (*page 56*)

22. [c] Stage 2

Stage 2: State of delirium or "excitement phase" begins when the patient loses consciousness and continues until stage 3. Respiration is irregular and breath holding is common. (*page 57*)

23. [c] Stage 3

Stage 3: State of surgical anesthesia extends from the onset of regular respiration until respiration ceases. The eyes become fixed and the intercostal muscles and diaphragm are paralyzed. (*page 57*)

24. [d] At the patient's side, prepared to assist the anesthesia care provider

During induction of general anesthesia, the circulating nurse should be at the patient's side. At all times, but especially at induction of general anesthesia, the nurse must keep all noise and activity in abeyance and should be prepared to hand the anesthesia care provider the endotracheal tube and make sure all suction attachments are functioning properly before induction. (*page 57*)

25. [c] Apply cricoid pressure

Cricoid pressure is applied with the thumb and first two digits. The cricoid cartilage is felt with the fingers immediately below the cricoid notch, and pressure is applied firmly on both sides of the midline. This effectively closes off the esophagus and allows better visualization of the vocal cords by the anesthetist. (*page 57*)

26. [a] Irritation of the larynx

If purely an inhalation anesthetic is used, induction is slower and the excitement phase is longer. A common problem is irritation of the larynx, resulting in coughing and laryngospasm. (*page 57*)

27. [a] Dim the lights

Ketamine may induce unpleasant dreams, and hallucinations are common after the procedure. Dimming of the lights as the patient emerges from anesthesia is recommended. (*page 57*)

28. [b] Hypoxia

Emergence from general anesthesia is often accompanied by shivering and agitation, especially in young patients. The most important consideration before restraining this type of patient is to rule out hypoxemia or serious changes in the vital signs. (*page 58*)

29. [d] Anesthesia provider

The anesthesia provider has the responsibility of undertaking transfusion only when other measures will no longer be effective in helping the patient cope with blood loss. To make a sound decision about transfusion and to quantitate the numbers and types of units, knowledge of blood loss is critical. (*page 58*)

30. [a] Rapid sequence induction

The induction of choice for patients undergoing emergency procedures is a rapid sequence induction, which involves intravenous agents, muscle relaxants, and the application of cricoid pressure. (*page 59*)

31. [d] Vomiting of stomach contents

Vomiting of stomach contents and subsequent aspiration is a real danger in emergency situations because the anesthesia evaluation of the patient may be brief, with little information available about whether and when the patient has eaten. (*page 59*)

32. [b] Malignant hyperthermia

Malignant hyperthermia is a hypermetabolic state that results in increased carbon dioxide production, oxygen consumption, and muscle membrane destruction. It is a rare inherited disorder and is characterized during the operative and invasive procedure by tachycardia, fever, acidosis, hyperkalemia, and myoglobinuria. (*page 59*)

33. [c] Succinylcholine

During the past 20 years, research has identified trigger agents for malignant hyperthermia, including succinylcholine and potent inhalation agents. (*page 59*)

34. [d] Dantrolene

Dantrolene sodium is the life-saving drug stocked near every area where anesthesia induction is performed, and a review of where this drug is kept is an important part of orientation. Because of the high cost of this medication, pharmacy departments often have a starter supply in the operative and invasive procedure suite and additional amounts in their central location. (*page 59*)

35. [c] Discontinuation of anesthesia

A common sequence of events when a malignant hyperthermia crisis happens is as follows: discontinue anesthesia, hyperventilate patient with 100% oxygen, request that the surgeon close quickly, request a malignant hyperthermia kit, request assistance from other anesthesia care providers. The anesthesia provider responsible for the case directs the team to mix and administer dantrolene, to cool the patient, to insert an indwelling catheter, and to obtain blood work. The team should be prepared for cardiac arrest. (*page 59*)

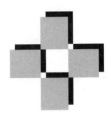

CHAPTER 5

Establishing and Maintaining a Sterile Field

Establishing and maintaining a sterile field concerns the patient care activities performed by the nurse and other members of the patient care team to create an operative or invasive procedure environment that minimizes the patient's risk for acquiring a nosocomial infection. The questions for this chapter will help the reader assess his or her knowledge about

- Identifying patients at risk for adverse outcomes related to establishing and maintaining a sterile field
- Donning operative attire
- Scrubbing the hands and arms
- Donning sterile gown and gloves
- Preparing the skin for the procedure
- Draping the patient and equipment

The reference used for this chapter is Phippen, M. L. & Wells, M. P. (1999). *Patient care during operative and invasive procedures.* Philadelphia: W. B. Saunders, pp. 61–93.

Questions

1. The patient's first line of defense against infection is:

   a. Flawless application of asepsis

   b. Intact skin

   c. New technologies

   d. Collective surgical conscience

2. How can wound infections be avoided during the operative or invasive procedure?

   a. Use of aseptic technique

   b. Prophylactic antibiotic therapy

   c. Collective surgical conscience

   d. Preoperative gastrointestinal cleansing

3. Which of the following statement is true regarding the definition of *sterile*?

   a. The condition of being free from all living organisms

   b. The act of vaporizing by heat, condensing, and collecting any volatilized products

   c. To make safe by removing or reducing contamination by infectious organisms or other harmful substances; the reduction of contamination to an acceptable level

   d. The process whereby heat is transmitted in a solid substance from molecule to molecule

4. In addition to ensuring accessibility of the operative site and preventing the transfer of microorganisms from the surgical team and the surrounding environment to the sterile field, the perioperative nurse:

   a. Ensures that the process of creating and maintaining the sterile field is accomplished in a cost-effective manner

   b. Uses disposable draping materials

   c. Does not adversely affect the patient's respiratory patterns, skin integrity, body temperature, or self-esteem

   d. Does not compromise the patient's skin integrity

5. Which of the following factors indicate that the patient is at high risk for wound infection?

    (1) Impaired skin integrity, impaired tissue integrity, and altered tissue perfusion

    (2) Increased hemoglobin concentration, leukopenia, and suppressed inflammatory response

    (3) Immunosuppression, inadequate acquired immunity, and existing infection

  a. 1 and 2

  b. 1 and 3

  c. 2 and 3

  d. All of the above

6. An obese patient with impaired tissue perfusion and poor skin turgor at the operative site is at high risk for:

  a. Impaired skin integrity, particularly around the operative site

  b. Injury during the operative procedure

  c. Altered skin integrity, particularly around the operative site

  d. Ineffective breathing patterns

7. Low body weight secondary to malnutrition, extremes in age, decreased metabolic rate, and the presence of medications causing vasodilation place the patient at risk for:

  a. Ineffective breathing patterns during the postoperative period

  b. Hyperthermia during the surgical procedure

  c. Impaired intraoperative body temperature

  d. Hypothermia during the surgical procedure

8. The surgical team is an environmental risk factor in the patient's potential for acquiring a postoperative wound infection. Properly worn surgical attire, gowns, and gloves:

  a. Prevent wound infection by acting as barriers to microorganisms that are shed from the skin, hair, and mucous membranes of members of the surgical team

  b. Attenuate the risk of microorganism shedding and spraying by placing a physical barrier between the patient and the surgical team, thereby reducing the amount of microorganisms introduced into the sterile field

  c. Prevent microorganism shedding and spraying by placing a physical barrier between the patient and the surgical team, thereby reducing the amount of microorganisms introduced into the sterile field

  d. Eliminate the surgical team as an environmental risk factor

9. Care must be taken by the perioperative nurse to ensure that the patient is not adversely affected, either physically or emotionally, by the process of creating and maintaining the sterile field. Specifically, a patient should remain free from:

    (1) Postoperative wound infection

    (2) Impaired skin integrity

    (3) Hyperthermia or hypothermia

    (4) Ineffective respiratory patterns

    (5) A disturbed self-esteem

  a. 1, 2, and 4

  b. 1, 2, and 5

  c. All of the above

  d. 1, 2, and 3

10. Select the statement that best describes the meaning of a surgical conscience.

  a. Surgical conscience involves a concept of self-inspection coupled with self-regulation and ethical commitment to maintaining the sterile field.

b. Surgical conscience involves a concept of self-inspection coupled with moral obligation, requires scientific and intellectual honesty, and is self-regulated in practice according to a deep personal commitment to the highest values.

c. Surgical conscience involves the concept of self-regulation, adherence to the Association of Operating Room Nurses (AORN) recommended practices for aseptic technique, and scientific and intellectual honesty.

d. Surgical conscience involves the concept of scientific and intellectual honesty and commitment to the highest values of perioperative nursing care.

11. *Sterile* is defined as being maximally free of all microorganisms. Perfect asepsis, however, is the absence of:

a. Disease-causing microorganisms and is an ideal toward which members of the surgical team should strive

b. Disease-causing microorganisms and is an ideal that members of the surgical team cannot achieve

c. Disease-causing microorganisms and is possible if all members of the surgical team wear operating room (OR) attire according to hospital policy and procedure

d. *All* exogenous microorganisms and is an ideal toward which members of the surgical team should strive

12. Sources of infection can be either endogenous or exogenous. Which statement is true?

a. Endogenous infection comes from the environment.

b. Endogenous infection comes from the large number of microorganisms found in and on the bodies of the patient and the team members.

c. Endogenous infection comes from body scurf of the surgical team members.

d. Endogenous infection comes from the patient, from the large number of microorganisms found in and on the body.

13. Donning proper surgical attire is a requirement for all personnel entering:

a. Operating rooms and the sterile core area of the surgical suite

b. Unrestricted, semirestricted, and restricted areas of the surgical suite

c. Restricted areas of the surgical suite

d. Semirestricted and restricted areas of the surgical suite

14. Team members with skin lesions:

a. May scrub if the lesion is treated with antibiotics and covered with an adhesive bandage

b. May scrub in emergencies if double gloved

c. Should not participate in direct patient care activities and should be prohibited in the restricted area of the surgical suite

d. May participate in direct patient care activities in the semirestricted area of the surgical suite if gloves are worn but should be prohibited in the restricted area of the surgical suite

15. Dressing properly for the OR requires:

a. Scrub top and pants that are easy to don and remove, a long-sleeved warm-up jacket for unscrubbed personnel, a disposable bouffant hat or hood, shoe covers, protective eyewear, and a disposable mask

b. Scrub top and pants that are easy to don and remove, a disposable bouffant hat or hood, shoe covers, protective eyewear, and a disposable mask

c. Scrub top and pants that are easy to don and remove, a long-sleeved warm-up jacket for unscrubbed personnel, a disposable bouffant hat or hood, protective eyewear, and a disposable mask

d. Scrub top and pants that are easy to don and remove, a long-sleeved warm-up jacket or surgical gown that ties at the waist for unscrubbed personnel, a disposable bouffant hat or hood, shoe covers, protective eyewear, and a disposable mask

16. Surgical masks are selected based on:

a. Comfort and nonallergenic properties

b. Protection they provide to the surgical team member from fluid splashed from the surgical field

c. Documented quality of microorganism filtration and comfort

d. Protection they provide the patient from aerosolization of microorganisms from the surgical team member

17. OR attire should be selected for proper fit because tight-fitting attire:

a. Does not present a professional image

b. Rubs against the body surfaces and increases the dispersal of body scurf into the surgical environment

c. Rubs against the body surfaces and may increase the dispersal of body scurf

d. Is uncomfortable to wear

18. Hair should be covered with a bouffant hat or hood before donning the scrub top:

a. To prevent the possible dispersal of microorganisms and scalp hair onto the scrub attire

b. To prevent hair from falling onto the back field

c. To protect the hair from fluid splashes

d. To protect the patient from dispersal of microorganisms and scalp hair onto the surgical wound

19. Disposable shoe covers should be worn during a surgical procedure:

a. To prevent contamination of the restricted area with debris tracked into the OR from other areas of the hospital

b. Because the restricted area is considered a sterile area

c. To prevent contamination of the sanitized OR floor with debris tracked into the OR from other areas of the hospital

d. To protect footwear from gross contamination

20. Which of the following statements concerning the wearing of a surgical mask is true?

a. A mask should be worn in the semi-restricted and restricted area of the surgical suite.

b. A surgical mask should be worn when one is entering areas such as the substerile area, the sterile center core, and the scrub sink area when team members are scrubbing.

c. After a contaminated case, the nurse should remove the mask by handling it by the strings only unless gloves are worn.

d. A mask should be changed every hour for best effectiveness.

21. Marge Williams is a 16-year-old scheduled for a breast biopsy. The patient has agreed to have the procedure done under a local anesthestic. This patient is at high risk for:

a. Hypothermia before and during the operative procedure

b. Impaired skin integrity

c. Self-esteem disturbance

d. Wound infection

22. How can the operative or invasive procedure team minimize the transmission of respiratory bacteria to the patient?

    a. Wear a properly fitted mask.

    b. Control body fluid splashes.

    c. Use standard precautions at all times.

    d. Have yearly *Staphylococcus* culturing done.

23. One objective of the surgical hand scrub is to:

    a. Destroy transient and resident microorganisms on the skin

    b. Leave an antimicrobial residue on the skin to prevent growth of microorganisms during the surgical procedure

    c. Remove gross contaminants, dirt, skin oil, and microbes from the skin

    d. Eliminate resident bacteria while reducing the transient colony count

24. There are two types of microorganisms present on the skin:

    a. Transient and resident

    b. Pathological and resident

    c. Nonresident and resident

    d. Migrant and resident

25. Scrubbing with an antimicrobial agent:

    a. Removes resident microorganisms from the skin

    b. Inhibits or kills resident microorganisms

    c. Prevents the transmission of resident microorganisms to the patient in the event that a surgical glove is torn or punctured during the procedure

    d. Inhibits or kills transient microorganisms

26. Transient microorganisms are:

    a. Attached to the skin at the base of hair follicles and are easily removed by vigorous scrubbing with a scrub brush

    b. Loosely attached to the skin surface and are easily removed by hand washing with an antimicrobial agent

    c. Loosely attached to the skin surface and are easily removed by hand washing with soap and water

    d. The primary cause of wound infections

27. Which statements are true?

    (1) When performed correctly, the anatomical timed scrub ensures sufficient exposure of all skin surfaces to friction and to an antimicrobial agent.

    (2) When performed correctly, the counted-brush-stroke scrub ensures sufficient exposure of all skin surfaces to friction and to an antimicrobial agent.

    (3) The anatomical timed scrub specifies a 10-minute scrub for the first case of the day.

    (4) The anatomical timed scrub specifies a 5-minute scrub for the first case of the day and a 3-minute scrub for all remaining cases that day.

    a. 1, 2, and 4

    b. 2 and 3

    c. 1 and 2

    d. 2

28. Which statement is true concerning antimicrobial agents for surgical scrubs?

    a. The antimicrobial agent selected for the surgical hand scrub should be broad-spectrum and capable of reducing and inhibiting both transient and resident microorganisms; be fast acting, easily applied, and able to maintain its effectiveness for several hours; be nonirritating and nonsensitizing; not be rendered ineffective by soaps, detergents, organic matter, or alcohol; and be approved by the US Food and Drug Administration (FDA)

b. The antimicrobial agent selected for the surgical hand scrub should be broad-spectrum and capable of killing both transient and resident microorganisms; be able to maintain its effectiveness for 4 hours; be nonirritating and nonsensitizing; be easily rinsed from the skin; not be rendered ineffective by soaps, detergents, organic matter, or alcohol; and be approved by the US FDA and the Association of Practitioners of Infection Control.

c. The antimicrobial agent selected for the surgical hand scrub should be broad-spectrum and capable of inhibiting both transient and resident microorganisms; have a cumulative effect after repeated applications; be able to maintain its effectiveness for 3 hours; be nonirritating and nonsensitizing; not be rendered ineffective by soaps, detergents, organic matter, or alcohol; and be approved by the AORN and the US FDA.

d. The antimicrobial agent selected for the surgical hand scrub should be broad-spectrum and capable of reducing the numbers of all microorganisms present on the skin; be nonstaining and able to maintain its effectiveness for 6 hours; be nonirritating and nonsensitizing; not be rendered ineffective by soaps, detergents, organic matter, or alcohol; and be approved by the US FDA and the Centers for Disease Control and Prevention.

29. What is the first step when scrubbing the hands and arms for the first scrub of the day?

a. Rinse the hands and arms thoroughly under running water to remove transient flora and gross contaminants.

b. Clean nails and cuticles under running water with the plastic nail stick.

c. Remove all jewelry.

d. Wash and rinse the hands for the initial wash with water and a small amount of antimicrobial agent to remove transient flora and gross contaminants.

30. One of the primary goals of the scrub process is to ensure that:

a. All surfaces of the hands and arms are sufficiently exposed to friction and an antimicrobial agent

b. Two scrub brushes are used

c. The correct amount of time is used to accomplish the scrub

d. A microbial agent with a high kill rate is used

31. The surgical team dons gowns and gloves to:

a. Protect the patient from cross-contamination

b. Protect the patient and themselves from cross-contamination

c. Protect themselves from cross-contamination

d. Prevent the transfer of pathogens from the surgical team to the patient

32. During unassisted gowning and gloving, the scrub person:

a. May don the gown and gloves from the back table if the gown and gloves were placed near the edge of the table and the scrub person does not reach over the sterile field

b. Should don the gown and gloves from the back table in an emergency

c. Should don the gown and gloves in a separate sterile area because of the possibility of water dripping off the arms and onto the sterile field

d. May don the gown and gloves from the back table if water is shaken from the arms before the OR is entered

33. When selecting gowns for a surgical procedure, the nurse considers:

a. Guidelines delineated in Occupational Safety and Health Association (OSHA) standards

b. Guidelines delineated in AORN-recommended practices

c. OSHA standards and AORN-recommended practices

d. The proposed surgery and the degree of blood and fluid splashing inherent in the procedure

34. Surgical gloves may be donned by either the closed-glove technique or the open-glove technique. Which of the following statements is true about the closed-glove technique?

a. The closed-glove technique prevents bare skin exposure during gowning and donning of sterile gloves, thereby lessening the chance of contamination.

b. The closed-glove technique should be used for regloving if the scrub person contaminates his or her gloves during the surgical procedure.

c. The closed-glove technique prevents bare skin exposure during gowning and donning of sterile gloves, thereby preventing contamination.

d. The closed-glove technique is preferred when donning sterile gloves for procedures that do not require sterile gowns.

35. When gowning a surgical team member, the scrub person protects his or her sterile gloves by:

a. Wearing a second pair of gloves

b. Identifying the armholes and placing the gown on the outstretched hands of the scrubbed team member

c. Forming a protective cuff by placing the hands at shoulder level on the exterior side of the gown and draping the gown over the gloves

d. Immediately releasing the gown once the team member has inserted his or her arms into the gown armholes

36. When a glove becomes contaminated, the scrub person has three options for re-gloving:

a. Ask for assistance from a sterile team member in regloving; remove gloves and reglove using the closed-glove method; apply a sterile glove over the contaminated glove.

b. Ask for assistance from a sterile team member in regloving; remove both gown and gloves and regown and reglove using the open-glove method; apply a sterile glove over the contaminated glove.

c. Ask for assistance from a sterile team member in regloving; remove both gown and gloves and regown and reglove; apply a sterile glove over the contaminated glove.

d. Ask for assistance from the circulating nurse in regloving; remove both gown and gloves and regown and reglove; apply a sterile glove over the contaminated glove.

37. Why is an antimicrobial residue left on the skin after the operative skin preparation?

a. Maintains the sterile surgical site

b. Inhibits rebound growth of microorganisms during the procedure

c. Acts as an additional barrier to microorganisms

d. Prevents transient microorganism migration to the sterile field

38. How is transient flora removed from the skin?

    a. Rubbed with an alcohol-based skin preparation

    b. Scrubbed with a degreaser

    c. Washed with soap and water

    d. Cannot be removed from the skin

39. Once the decision is made to shave the skin, when should shaving take place?

    a. Immediately before the procedure

    b. The night before the procedure

    c. At the physician's office the morning of the procedure

    d. At the convenience of the patient

40. What is the direct effect between the time of shaving and the start of the procedure?

    a. Microbial count increases

    b. Wound infection rate increases

    c. Microbial count decreases

    d. Wound infection rate decreases

41. Aseptic technique is practiced to:

    a. Prevent contamination of the open wound with pathogenic microorganisms

    b. Isolate the operative site from the surrounding nonsterile physical environment

    c. Create a sterile field in which surgery can be performed safely

    d. Lessen the need for intraoperative antibiotics

42. The sterile field consists of:

    a. The draped patient's body around the site of the incision, the Mayo stand, the back table, the ring stand, and any other furniture or equipment covered with sterile drapes

    b. The Mayo stand, the back table, the ring stand, and any other furniture or equipment covered with sterile drapes as well as any surgical team member wearing sterile surgical attire

    c. The draped patient's body around the site of the incision, the Mayo stand, the back table, the ring stand, and any surgical team member wearing sterile surgical attire

    d. The draped patient's body around the incision site, the Mayo stand, the back table, the ring stand, and any other furniture or equipment covered with sterile drapes, as well as any surgical team member wearing sterile surgical attire

43. How can the operative-invasive procedure nurse prevent strike-through?

    a. Use impervious drapes

    b. Practice standard precautions

    c. Involve the physician in the draping process

    d. Limit the amount of solutions added to the sterile field

✚ Answers

1. [b] Intact skin

   Skin is the patient's first line of defense against infection. Disruption of the skin surface from an operative incision or trauma compromises that line of defense by creating an entry for microorganisms. (*page 61*)

2. [a] Use of aseptic technique

   Preventing wound infection requires the flawless application of aseptic technique by all members of the patient care team. (*page 61*)

3. [a] The condition of being free from all living organisms

   Sterile is defined as being maximally free of all microorganisms. Perfect asepsis, the absence of disease-causing microorganism, is the ideal toward which team members should strive. (*page 61*)

4. [c] Does not adversely affect the patient's respiratory patterns, skin integrity, body temperature, or self-esteem

In addition to ensuring accessibility of the operative site and preventing the transfer of microorganisms from the surgical team and the surrounding environment to the sterile field, the perioperative nurse does not adversely affect the patient's respiratory patterns, skin integrity, body temperature, or self-esteem. This is demonstrated by the patient's remaining free from wound infection, impaired skin integrity, hypothermia, and ineffective breathing patterns. (*page 63*)

5. [b] 1 and 3

The presence of impaired skin integrity, impaired tissue integrity, altered tissue perfusion, immunosuppression, inadequate acquired immunity, and existing infection greatly increases the patient's risk for postoperative wound infection. (*page 64*)

6. [a] Impaired skin integrity, particularly around the operative site

An obese patient with impaired tissue perfusion and poor skin turgor at the operative site is at high risk for impaired skin integrity, particularly around the operative site. (*page 64*)

7. [d] Hypothermia during the surgical procedure

Low body weight secondary to malnutrition, extremes in age, decreased metabolic rate, and the use of medications causing vasodilation place the patient at risk for hypothermia during the surgical procedure. (*page 64*)

8. [b] Attenuate the risk of microorganism shedding and spraying by placing a physical barrier between the patient and the surgical team, thereby reducing the amount of microorganisms introduced into the sterile field

The surgical team is an environmental risk factor in the patient's potential for acquiring a postoperative wound infection. Properly worn surgical attire, gowns, and gloves attenuate the risk of microorganism shedding and spraying by placing a physical barrier between the patient and the surgical team, which reduces the amount of microorganisms introduced into the sterile field. (*page 64*)

9. [c] All of the above

Care must be taken by the perioperative nurse to ensure that the patient is not adversely affected, either physically or emotionally, by the process of creating and maintaining the sterile field. Specifically, a patient should remain free from postoperative wound infection, impaired skin integrity, hyperthermia or hypothermia, ineffective respiratory patterns, and disturbed self-esteem. (*page 64*)

10. [b] Surgical conscience involves a concept of self-inspection coupled with moral obligation, requires scientific and intellectual honesty, and is self-regulated in practice according to a deep personal commitment to the highest values.

All team members must maintain both an individual and collective surgical conscience. A surgical conscience involves a concept of self-inspection coupled with moral obligation, requires scientific and intellectual honesty, and is self-regulated in practice according to a deep personal commitment to the highest values. (*page 61*)

11. [a] Disease causing microorganisms and is an ideal toward which members of the surgical team should strive

Sterile is defined as being maximally free of all microorganisms. Perfect asepsis is the absence of disease-causing microorganisms and is an ideal toward which members of the surgical team should strive. (*page 61*)

12. [d] Endogenous infections come from the patient, from the large number of microorganisms found in and on the body.

Exogenous infections are acquired from organisms outside the patient's body. (*page 61*)

13. [d] Semirestricted and restricted areas of the surgical suite

All personnel entering the semirestricted and restricted patient areas of the operative suite must wear proper operative attire. While in semirestricted areas, personnel wear operative attire and head gear that covers all head and facial hair. In the restricted areas, in addition to operative attire, personnel wear masks if open sterile instruments, supplies, equipment, or scrubbed personnel are present. (*page 62*)

14. [c] Should not participate in direct patient care activities and should be prohibited in the restricted area of the surgical suite

Team members with an infectious disease, such as an upper respiratory tract illness, or with skin lesions, boils, or infected lesions should neither participate in direct patient care activities nor work in the restricted area of the operative-invasive procedure suite. (*page 62*)

15. [a] Scrub top and pants that are easy to don and remove, a long-sleeved warm-up jacket for unscrubbed personnel, a disposable bouffant hat or hood, shoe covers, protective eyewear, and a disposable mask

When dressing for a restricted or semirestricted area, one should wear a scrub top and pants that are easy to don and remove, a long sleeved warm-up jacket if unscrubbed (to minimize shedding from bare arms), a disposable bouffant hat or hood, shoe covers (optional), protective eyewear, and a disposable mask. (*page 62*)

16. [c] Documented quality of microorganism filtration and comfort

Surgical masks are selected based on the documented quality of microorganism filtration and comfort. An acceptable mask has at least a 95% efficiency rating. (*page 62*)

17. [c] Rubs against the body surfaces and may increase the dispersal of body scurf

OR attire should be selected for proper fit because tight-fitting OR attire rubs against the body surfaces and may increase the dispersal of body scurf. (*page 62*)

18. [a] To prevent the possible dispersal of microorganisms and scalp hair onto the scrub attire

To prevent the possible dispersal of microorganisms and scalp hair onto the scrub attire, the hair should be covered with a bouffant hat or hood before the scrub top is donned. The hat or hood is adjusted to cover all scalp hair. (*page 62*)

19. [d] To protect footwear from gross contamination

When contamination of footwear with blood and body fluids is a risk, disposable shoe covers are worn to protect footwear from gross contamination. Shoe covers that become moist or contaminated with body fluids or tissue must be removed before leaving the room. (*page 62*)

20. [b] A surgical mask should be worn when one is entering areas such as the substerile area, the sterile center core, and the scrub sink area when team members are scrubbing.

When one is entering areas such as the substerile area, the sterile center core, and the scrub sink area when team members are scrubbing, a surgical mask should be worn. (*page 62*)

21. [c] Self-esteem disturbance

Risk factors associated with the nursing diagnosis *Risk for Self-Esteem Disturbance* include cultural or religious beliefs (prohibitions against nudity in the presence of the opposite sex); location of the operative procedure site, such as genitalia or breast for female patients; consciousness during the procedure; mixed gender of the staff; and unnecessary traffic flow in the operative and invasive procedure suite. (*page 64*)

22. [a] Wear a properly fitted mask.

A properly applied mask minimizes the transmission of nasopharyngeal and respiratory bacteria from the patient care team to the patient. The mask should be changed between procedures. (*page 66*)

23. [c] Remove gross contamination, dirt, skin oil, and microbes from the skin

The objectives of the surgical hand scrub are to remove gross contaminants, dirt, skin oil, and microbes from the skin; to eliminate transient bacteria while reducing the resident colony count; and to leave an antimicrobial residue on the skin to inhibit the regrowth of microorganisms. (*page 66*)

24. [a] Transient and resident

Two types of microorganisms are present on the skin—transient microorganisms, which are loosely attached to the skin surface, and resident microorganisms, which survive and multiply in superficial skin layers and hair follicles and which can cause wound infection when allowed to enter deep tissue during the procedure. (*page 67*)

25. [b] Inhibits or kills resident microorganisms

Scrubbing with an antimicrobial agent inhibits or kills resident microorganisms. (*page 67*)

26. [b] Loosely attached to the skin surface and are easily removed by hand washing with an antimicrobial agent

Transient microorganisms are loosely attached to the skin surface and can be easily removed by hand washing with soap and water. (*page 67*)

27. [c] 1 and 2

When performed correctly, both the anatomical timed scrub and the counted-brush-stroke ensure sufficient exposure of all skin surfaces to friction and to an antimicrobial agent. The anatomical timed scrub specifies a prescribed amount of time for each anatomical area. The counted-brush-stroke denotes a set number of brush strokes to each surface of the fingers, hands, and forearms. (*page 67*)

28. [a] The antimicrobial agent selected for the surgical hand scrub should be broad

spectrum and capable of reducing and inhibiting both transient and resident microorganisms; be fast acting, easily applied, and able to maintain effectiveness for several hours; be nonirritating and nonsensitizing; not be rendered ineffective by soaps, detergents, organic matter, or alcohol; and be approved by the US FDA.

The antimicrobial agent selected for the surgical hand scrub should be broad spectrum and capable of reducing and inhibiting both transient and resident microorganisms; be fast acting, easily applied, and able to maintain its effectiveness for several hours; be nonirritating and nonsensitizing; not be rendered ineffective by soaps, detergents, organic matter, or alcohol; and be approved by the US FDA. (*page 67*)

29. [c] Remove all jewelry

One must examine the hands and forearms for good skin integrity and remove all jewelry before the first scrub of the day. Nails should be short and free from chipped and cracked polish; cuticles should be in good condition. (*page 67*)

30. [a] All surfaces of the hands and arms are sufficiently exposed to friction and an antimicrobial agent

One of the primary goals of the scrub process is to ensure that all surfaces of the hands and arms are sufficiently exposed to friction and an antimicrobial agent. (*page 67*)

31. [b] Protect the patient and themselves from cross-contamination

The patient care team members don gowns and gloves to protect the patient and themselves from cross-contamination. Gloves and gowns provide a barrier and prevent the transfer of microorganisms from the skin and clothing to the incision. (*page 70*)

32. [c] Should don the sterile gown and gloves in a separate sterile area because of the possibility of water dripping off the arms and onto the sterile field

When donning unassisted gowning and gloving, one must do so from a separate sterile surface because the water may drip off the arms and onto the sterile field, contaminating it. (*page 70*)

33. [d] The proposed surgery and the degree of blood and fluid splashing inherent in the procedure

When selecting gowns for a surgical procedure, the nurse considers the proposed surgery and the degree of blood and fluid splashing inherent in the procedure. (*page 71*)

34. [a] The closed-glove technique prevents bare skin exposure during gowning and donning of sterile gloves, thereby lessening the chance of contamination.

The open-glove technique should be used only when donning gloves for procedures that do not require sterile gloves. (*page 71*)

35. [c] Form a protective cuff by placing the hands at shoulder level on the exterior side of the gown and draping the gown over the gloves

When gowning a surgical team member, the scrub person protects his or her sterile gloves by forming a protective cuff by placing the hands at shoulder level exterior side of the gown and draping the gown over the gloves. (*page 76*)

36. [c] Ask for assistance from a sterile team member in regloving; remove both gown and gloves and regown and reglove; apply a sterile glove over the contaminated glove.

When a glove becomes contaminated, the scrub person should ask for assistance from a sterile team member in regloving, or remove both gown and gloves and regown and reglove, or apply a sterile glove over the contaminated glove. (*page 77*)

37. [b] Inhibits rebound growth of microorganisms during the procedure

An antimicrobial residue should be left on the skin to inhibit rebound growth of microorganisms during the procedure. (*page 77*)

38. [c] Washed with soap and water

Transient flora reside on the epidermis and are easily removed with soap and water. (*page 77*)

39. [a] Immediately before the procedure

Hair should not be removed unless it interferes with the incision. If shaving is deemed necessary, it is performed immediately before the procedure. (*page 78*)

40. [b] Wound infection rate increases

The time between shaving and the procedure has a direct effect on wound infection rate: the longer the delay between the shave and the procedure, the greater the risk of postprocedure infection. (*page 78*)

41. [b] Isolate the operative site from the surrounding nonsterile physical environment

The primary functions of draping the patient and equipment are to define and establish the sterile field during the operative or invasive procedure by isolating the incision site and to prevent microbial migration from nonsterile to sterile areas. (*page 84*)

42. [d] The draped patient's body around the incision site, the Mayo stand, the back table, the ring stand, and any other furniture or equipment covered with sterile drapes, as well as a surgical team member wearing sterile surgical attire

The area draped includes the patient; the area from the anesthesia screen and armboards to the foot of the bed; the patient care team in sterile attire; and the Mayo stand, back table, ring stand, and any other equipment used during the procedure.(*page 84*)

43. [a] Use impervious drapes

Strike-through is prevented by use of an impervious, fluid-proof fabric. (*page 85*)

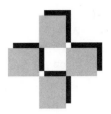

CHAPTER 6

Performing Sponge, Sharp, and Instrument Counts

Performing sponge, sharp, and instrument counts describes the patient care activity that accounts for items to ensure that they are not retained in the operative wound after closure. This crucial activity is an integral component of safe patient care during operative and invasive procedures. The questions for this chapter will help the reader assess his or her knowledge about

• Identifying the patient's risk for adverse outcomes related to the retention of foreign bodies
• Initiating count procedures that reduce the patient's risk for retained foreign bodies
• Initiating incorrect count procedures
• Documenting the count results according to facility policy and procedures

The reference used for this chapter is Phippen, M. L., & Wells, M. P. (1999). *Patient care during operative and invasive procedures.* Philadelphia: W. B. Saunders, pp. 94–96.

✚ Questions

1. Members of the operative nursing team are responsible for taking the measures necessary to provide safe patient care. Which statement is true concerning safe patient care as it relates to sponge, sharp, and instrument counts?

   a. The nurse, functioning as the circulator, ensures that the Association of Operating Room Nurses (AORN) Recommended Practices for Sponge, Sharp, and Instruments Counts are implemented for every case.

   b. The nurse, functioning as the scrub person, ensures that the AORN Recommended Practices for Sponge, Sharp, and Instruments Counts are implemented according to operating room policy and procedure.

   c. The nurse, functioning as the circulator, ensures that the appropriate counting policies and procedures are implemented.

   d. The scrub person collaborates with the surgeon in accounting for all sponges, sharps, and instruments.

2. AORN Recommended Practices for Sponge, Sharp, and Instrument Counts:

   a. Serve as the national standard for performing sponge, sharp, and instrument counts

   b. Provide guidelines for the development of institutional policies and procedures for performing sponge, sharp, and instrument counts

   c. State that the registered nurse is held liable if the patient has a retained sponge, sharp, or instrument following surgery

   d. Promote a minimal level of practice for performing sponge, sharp, and instrument counts

3. AORN Recommended Practices for Sponge, Sharp, and Instrument Counts state that "instruments should be counted on all procedures in which the likelihood exists that an instrument could be retained" (1993). Because of this statement, hospitals are:

   a. Mandated to count instruments on all procedures

b. Legally required to count instruments on all procedures

c. Advised to count instruments on all procedures

d. Legally required to count instruments only on open-cavity surgical procedures

4. Instruments should be counted:

a. For all surgical procedures

b. For abdominal and thoracic procedures

c. For abdominal, thoracic, and hip procedures

d. According to institutional policy and procedure

5. A sponge, sharp, and instrument count policy should:

a. Provide direction for discontinuing counts; establish authority, responsibility, and accountability for sponge, sharp, and instrument counts; and provide protocols for incorrect counts

b. Provide direction for performing counts; provide direction for discontinuing counts; and provide protocols for incorrect counts

c. Establish authority, responsibility, and accountability for sponge, sharp, and instrument counts; mandate protocols for performing counts; provide direction for discontinuing counts; and provide protocols for incorrect counts

d. Establish authority, responsibility, and accountability for sponge, sharp, and instrument counts; provide direction for performing counts; provide direction for discontinuing counts; and provide protocols for incorrect counts

6. When institutional policies and procedures do not comply to the letter with AORN Recommended Practices for Sponge, Sharp, and Instrument Counts, legally, the nurse must:

a. Follow AORN Recommended Practices for Sponge, Sharp, and Instrument Counts

b. Know and carry out institutional policies and procedures

c. State in writing to administration that institutional policies and procedures for sponge, sharp, and instrument counts do not comply with AORN recommended practices and then comply with institutional policy and procedure

d. Report the institution to the state Board of Health

7. Accountability for sponges, sharps, and instruments is the primary responsibility of the:

a. First assistant and scrub person

b. Scrub person

c. Nurse

d. Surgeon and scrub person

8. If a sponge, sharp, or instrument is left in a patient and the patient sues and the suit goes to trial, the jury will determine:

a. That the nurse is guilty of negligence if AORN Recommended Practices for Sponge, Sharp, and Instrument Counts were not followed

b. That the nurse is guilty of negligence if institutional policies and procedures for sponge, sharp, and instrument counts were not followed

c. Whether the nurse did what any reasonable and prudent nurse would have done to account for the item before closure of the surgical wound

d. That the nurse is not accountable for the retained item if institutional policies and procedures for sponge, sharp, and instrument counts were followed

9. When deciding a lawsuit concerning a retained foreign body, the jury bases its decision on:

   a. Evidence presented at the trial, AORN recommended practices, state Board of Health regulations, and institutional policies and procedures

   b. Evidence presented at the trial, AORN recommended practices, Joint Commission on Accreditation of Healthcare Organizations guidelines, and institutional policies and procedures

   c. Evidence presented at the trial, AORN recommended practices, and institutional policies and procedures

   d. Testimony of the surgeon, AORN recommended practices, and institutional policies and procedures

10. *The patient is free from injury related to the retention of sponges, sharps, or instruments* is an example for an outcome standard associated with the nursing diagnosis of *High Risk for Injury related to retained foreign bodies.* Which of the following criteria *best* measure achievement of this outcome standard?

    a. Absence of abscess formation in the abdominal, retroperitoneal, and chest cavities; no sign of retained sponges, sharps, or instruments on postprocedure x-ray films

    b. Absence of unexplained pain, cramping, and fever; absence of abscess formation in the abdominal, retroperitoneal, and chest cavities; no sign of retained sponges, sharps, or instruments on postprocedure x-ray films

    c. Absence of unexplained pain, cramping, and fever; no sign of retained sponges, sharps, or instruments on postprocedure x-ray films

    d. Absence of unexplained pain, cramping, and fever; absence of abscess formation in the abdominal, retroperitoneal, and chest cavities

11. Sponges, sharps, and instruments should be counted before the beginning of the procedure, at the change of personnel, when sponges are added to the sterile field, before the closure of a deep or large incision or body cavity, and immediately before the completion of the procedure. When counting sponges, sharps, and instruments, the circulating nurse:

    a. Counts out loud

    b. Counts silently with the scrub person

    c. Counts out loud with the scrub person

    d. Counts quietly to avoid disturbing the patient

12. The scrub person should:

    a. Completely separate all sponges when counting

    b. Completely separate sponges if the circulating nurse is not close to the sterile field

    c. Completely separate laparotomy sponges when counting

    d. Not need to separate sponges if the circulating nurse is close to the sterile field and can clearly see the scrub person fanning the sponges

13. If a package of medium laparotomy sponges contains an additional sponge the scrub person should:

    a. Pass the extra sponge off the sterile field

    b. Pass the entire package of sponges off the sterile field

    c. Tell the circulating nurse to add the additional sponge to the count record

    d. Call the supervisor

14. During a procedure, five packages of suture with needles are added to the sterile field. When the packages are added, the scrub person:

    a. Opens all packages and counts the needles with the circulating nurse

b. Counts the number of needles indicated on the outside of the package; when the package is open, the scrub person verifies the number with the circulating nurse

c. And circulating nurse count the needles according to the number indicated on the package and then verify the number of needles when the package is opened

d. And circulating nurse count the needles according to the number indicated on the package, and then the scrub person verifies the number of needles with the first assistant or surgeon when the package is opened

15. When passing needles to the surgeon, the scrub person passes:

a. Each needle on an exchange basis

b. As many needles as required and mentally makes a note of the number of needles the surgeon has at the operative site

c. As many needles as required and asks the circulating nurse to document the number of needles the surgeon has at the operative site

d. Needles as requested by the surgeon

16. The nurse identifies patients at high risk for injury related to retained foreign bodies by assessing the patient for the presence of risk factors. Which factors place the patient at risk for injury related to retained foreign bodies?

a. Emergency surgery, hemorrhage, change of staff during the procedure, advanced age, obesity

b. Lenient institutional count policies and procedures, lengthy surgical procedure, emergency surgery, emaciation

c. Emergency surgery, hemorrhage, abdominal or thoracic surgery

d. Emergency surgery, hemorrhage, surgery that entails packing cavities

with sponges, change of nursing staff during the procedure, and lenient institutional count policies

17. If a needle is broken during a procedure, the first thing the scrub person and circulating nurse should do is:

a. Account for all pieces of the broken needle

b. Initiate an incident report

c. Alert the supervisor that a needle has been broken

d. Take a needle count

18. In the event of an incorrect count, the circulating nurse:

a. Alerts the supervisor

b. Orders an x-ray film

c. Alerts the surgeon and then recounts

d. Recounts and then notifies the surgeon if the item cannot be found during the recount

19. If a missing item is not found after a recount, the circulating nurse should:

a. Alert the supervisor

b. Ask the surgeon to explore the wound

c. Ask the surgeon to explore the wound; the nurse then looks in areas where the item could be concealed

d. Alert risk management

20. When documenting a count:

a. The circulating nurse and scrub person sign the operative record

b. Only the circulating nurse signs the operative record

c. The circulating nurse and scrub person follow AORN Recommended Practices for Sponge, Sharp, and Instrument Counts

d. The circulating nurse and scrub person follow institutional policy and procedure

21. According to AORN recommended practices, in the event of an incorrect count:

a. Never document the incorrect count in the operative record

b. Document the incorrect count only on incident reports

c. Document the actions taken

d. Document the incorrect count in the operative record

✠ Answers

1. [c] The nurse, functioning as the circulator, ensures that the appropriate count policies and procedures are implemented.

The nurse, functioning as the circulator, ensures that the AORN Recommended Practices for Sponge, Sharp, and Instruments Counts are implemented according to operating room policy and procedure. The duties of scrub person do not allow the amount of attention that is necessary to account for sponges, sharps, and instruments during a surgical procedure. (*page 94*)

2. [b] Provide guidelines for the development of institutional policies and procedures for performing sponge, sharp, and instrument counts

The AORN Recommended Practices for Sponge, Sharp, and Instrument Counts provides guidelines for the development of institutional policies and procedures for performing sponge, sharp, and instrument counts. The AORN recommended practices promote an optimal level of practice. (*page 94*)

3. [c] Advised to count instruments on all procedures

Healthcare facilities are advised to count instruments on all procedures. This recommended practice enables the facility to define what types of procedures require instrument counts. (*page 94*)

4. [d] According to institutional policy and procedure

The nurse counts instruments according to institutional policy and procedure. Institutional policy may direct counting instruments for all procedures or delineate the type of cases or circumstances that require an instrument count. (*page 94*)

5. [d] Establish authority, responsibility, and accountability for sponge, sharp, and instrument counts; provide direction for performing counts; provide direction for discontinuing counts; and provide protocols for incorrect counts.

According to AORN recommended practices, institutional policies and procedures establish authority, responsibility, and accountability for sponge, sharp, and instrument counts; provide direction for performing counts; provide direction for discontinuing counts; and provide protocols for incorrect counts. (*page 94*)

6. [b] Know and carry out institutional policies and procedures

When institutional policies and procedures do not comply to the letter with AORN Recommended Practices for Sponge, Sharp, and Instrument Counts, legally, the nurse must know and carry out institutional policies and procedures. AORN recommended practices promote an optimal level of practice; they have no authority to bind actual institutional practice. (*page 94*)

7. [c] Nurse

The nurse has primary responsibility for accountability of sponges, sharps, and instruments. (*page 94*)

8. [c] Whether the nurse did what any reasonable and prudent nurse would have done to account for the item before closure of the surgical wound.

The jury will determine whether the nurse did what any reasonable and prudent nurse would have done to account for the item before the surgical wound was closed in the event that a sponge, sharp, or instrument is left in a patient, the patient sues, and the suit goes to trial. (*page 94*)

9. [c] Evidence presented at the trial, AORN recommended practices, and institutional policies and procedures

Jury members will be instructed to base their decision on the evidence presented at the trial, such as expert witness testimony, AORN recommended practices, and institutional policies and procedures. Retained sponges, sharps, and instruments may result in a verdict of negligence against the nurse. (*page 94*)

10. [b] Absence of unexplained pain, cramping, and fever; absence of abscess formation in the abdominal, retroperitoneal, and chest cavities; no sign of retained sponges, sharps, or instruments on postprocedure x-ray films

Absence of unexplained pain, cramping, and fever; absence of abscess formation in the abdominal, retroperitoneal, and chest cavities; and no sign of retained sponges, sharps, or instruments of postprocedure x-ray films are examples of criteria to measure if a patient is free from injury related to the retention of sponges, sharps, or instruments. (*page 95*)

11. [c] Counts out loud with the scrub person

When counting sponges, sharps, and instruments, the circulating nurse counts out loud with the scrub person. Counting silently may lead to errors. Counting out loud verifies between the circulating nurse and scrub the number of counted items on the sterile field. (*page 95*)

12. [a] Completely separate all sponges when counting

The scrub person should completely separate sponges when counting. Errors can occur in prepackaged sponges. Separating the sponges ensures that an extra folded sponge is not hidden from view in the bundle of sponges. (*page 95*)

13. [b] Pass the entire package of sponges off the sterile field

Packages of sponges that contain more or fewer than the number of sponges indicated on the package should be passed off the sterile field. Correcting the discrepancy by removing the extra sponge or adjusting the number of sponges on the count record may lead to errors when sponges are counted at the end of the procedure. (*page 95*)

14. [c] And circulating nurse count the needles according to the number indicated on the package and then verify the number of needles when the package is opened

When packages of suture with attached needles are added to the sterile field, the scrub person and circulating nurse count the needles according to the number indicated on the package and then verify the number of needles when the package is opened. (*page 95*)

15. [a] Each needle on an exchange basis

When passing needles to the surgeon, the scrub person passes each needle on an exchange basis. This enables the scrub person to maintain control of the number of needles at the operative site. (*page 95*)

16. [d] Emergency surgery, hemorrhage, surgery that entails packing cavities with sponges, change of nursing staff during the procedure, and lenient institutional count policies

Emergency surgery, hemorrhage, surgery that entails packing cavities with sponges, change of nursing staff during the procedure, and lenient institutional count policies place the patient at risk for injury related to retained foreign bodies. (*page 95*)

17. [a] Account for all pieces of the broken needle

The circulating nurse and scrub person must account for all pieces of broken needle to ensure that pieces are not inadvertently left in the patient at closure. (*page 95*)

18. [c] Alerts the surgeon and then recounts

If a counted item cannot be found, the circulating nurse first alerts the surgeon and then begins a recount. This provides the surgeon with the option of searching the operative site before closing the wound. (*page 96*)

19. [c] Ask the surgeon to explore the wound; the nurse then looks in areas where the item could be concealed

If a missing item is not found after a recount, the circulating nurse should ask the surgeon to explore the wound. The nurse looks in areas where the item could be concealed. (*page 96*)

20. [d] The circulating nurse and scrub person follow institutional policy and procedures

According to the AORN Recommended Practices for Sponge, Sharp, and Instrument Counts, the circulating nurse and scrub person follow institutional policy and procedure when documenting a count. (*page 96*)

21. [c] Document the actions taken

According to AORN recommended practices, in the event of an incorrect count, the nurse documents the actions taken. The nurse follows institutional policies and procedures when documenting actions taken in response to incorrect counts. (*page 96*)

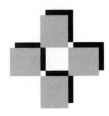

CHAPTER 7

Providing Instruments, Equipment, and Supplies

The nurse provides instruments, equipment, and supplies to assist in the provision of safe patient care and to enable the physician to effectively perform an operative or invasive procedure. The questions for this chapter will help the reader assess his or her knowledge about

- Identifying patients at risk for adverse outcomes related to providing instruments, equipment, and supplies
- Selecting instruments, equipment, supplies, and sutures for an operative or invasive procedure
- Delivering instruments, supplies, and sutures to the sterile field
- Arranging instruments and supplies on the instrument table and Mayo tray
- Passing instruments and supplies to the physician
- Preparing and passing sutures to the physician
- Preparing patient warming systems for use
- Applying and removing a pneumatic tourniquet
- Preparing air-powered instruments for use
- Preparing electrical instruments and equipment for use
- Implementing electrosurgical safety precautions
- Applying dressings
- Assisting with the application of casts and splints
- Preparing and operating endoscopic equipment

The reference used for this chapter is Phippen, M. L., & Wells, M. P. (1999). *Patient care during operative and invasive procedures.* Philadelphia: W. B. Saunders, pp. 97–111.

Questions

1. It is the goal of the operative and invasive procedure nurse to have all instrumentation, supplies, and equipment available and functioning to prevent:

   a. Extended anesthesia time

   b. Nosocomial infections

   c. Patient injury

   d. Delay of surgical schedule

2. Which statement is true concerning sterile packages?

   a. Commercially prepared items are the only sterile items that must have an expiration date listed on the package before the operative or invasive procedure nurse presents them to the sterile field.

   b. If the sterile setup has been open but not immediately used, the operative or invasive procedure nurse should cover the setup with a cloth sheet or other protective material and label it with the surgeon's name.

   c. The operative and invasive procedure nurse may not delegate the responsibility of providing instruments, equipment, or supplies to an unlicensed or assistive person.

   d. Compromise of the package compromises sterility.

3. Risk factors associated with altered body temperature during surgery are:

   a. Internal and external metal prosthetic devices

b. Scar tissue and high white blood cell counts

c. High white blood cell counts and internal metal prosthetics

d. Type of anesthesia, cold room, and decreased body fat

4. The appropriate method of introducing a heavy object to the sterile field is to:

a. Flip the item onto the Mayo stand

b. Flip the item onto the back table

c. Open the item on a separate table

d. Don sterile gloves and hand the item to scrub person

5. After pouring the sterile water into a basin on the back table, 100 mL of water remains in the bottle. The appropriate action for the circulating nurse would be to:

a. Recap the bottle and add remaining solution later in the procedure

b. Do not recap, but save the remaining solution for later in the case

c. Recap and save the remaining solution for cleanup of blood or body fluid spills during the procedure

d. Discard the unused portion of solution

6. To avoid puncturing sterile gloves when working with instruments, the scrub person will:

a. Arrange clamps according to order of use

b. Double glove

c. Close towel clip box locks

d. Use towel rolls

7. The outcome standard *The patient is free from injury related to provision of instruments during surgery* will be demonstrated by no evidence of:

a. Alterations in temperature or electrical injury

b. Burns or necrosis of the skin

c. Nosocomial infection or upper respiratory tract infection

d. Skin cool to the touch or skin abrasions

8. Risk factors associated with high risk for injury related to use of electrical equipment during surgery include:

a. Scar tissue, type of anesthesia

b. Wrinkled padding, cold room temperature

c. Excessive hair, pacemaker

d. Excessive sedation, pooling of preparation solution

9. Failure of the sterilization or disinfection process is a risk factor for high risk for:

a. Injury related to electrical equipment

b. Injury related to pneumatic tourniquet

c. Infection

d. Altered body temperature

10. Risk factors associated with the high risk for infection include:

a. Use of faulty equipment

b. Inadequate secondary defenses

c. Use of unwarmed irrigation solution

d. Cold room temperature

11. In patients free from injury related to pneumatic tourniquet use, there is no evidence of:

a. Chemical burns or nerve damage

b. Bruising, blisters, altered cardiac output

c. Chemical burns or urinary tract infection

d. Cool skin or shivering

12. The patient is free from electrical equipment related injury, as evidenced by no:

    a. Urinary tract infection

    b. Alteration in tissue perfusion

    c. Skin abrasions or swelling

    d. Shivering

13. No evidence of shivering, chattering of teeth, or cool skin is the expected outcome for the outcome standard:

    a. *Patient's body temperature maintained within normal limits*

    b. *Patient is free from nosocomial infection*

    c. *Patient is free from injury related to equipment*

    d. *Patient is free from injury related to pneumatic cuff*

14. Improper tourniquet cuff size, wrinkled padding, and pooling of preparation solution under the cuff are all risk factors associated with high risk for:

    a. Injury related to electrical equipment

    b. Infection

    c. Altered body temperature

    d. Injury related to use of pneumatic tourniquet

15. Risk factors associated with hypothermia include:

    a. Elevated white blood cell count

    b. Hypothyroidism

    c. History of smoking

    d. Use of flammable prep solutions

16. Inaccurate and outdated physician preference cards are a risk factor for:

    a. Injury related to extended anesthesia time

    b. Risk for hyperthermia

    c. Risk for nosocomial infection

    d. Injury related to electrical instrumentation

17. *The patient is free from bruising, blisters, pinching, or necrosis of the skin* is the expected outcome for:

    a. Patient is free from nosocomial infections

    b. Patient is free from injury related to increased anesthesia time

    c. Patient is free from injury related to pneumatic tourniquet use

    d. Patient is free from injury related to electrical instrument use

18. A wrapped item should be positioned so that the top flap is opened:

    a. Away from the body

    b. Toward the body

    c. To the left

    d. To the right

19. When opening a peel-back package, if the scrub nurse cannot accept the sterile item, the circulating nurse should:

    a. Open the item on an appropriate-sized table

    b. Flip items onto sterile field

    c. Wait until scrub nurse can receive the package

    d. Offer the sterile item to any member of the sterile team

20. A cloth-wrapped package should not be used if:

    a. It weighs more than 10 lb

    b. It has been stored in central supply for more than 10 days

    c. It has been gas sterilized

    d. It has been dropped on the floor

21. What instrument is used to assist the scrub nurse with placing the blade on the scalpel handle?

    a. Needle holder

    b. Kocher

    c. Crile

    d. Peon

22. To facilitate continuity of care during staff changes, back tables should be:

    a. Kept at the right of the operating room (OR) bed

    b. Kept blood free

    c. Individualized for physician preference

    d. Uniformly set up

23. The scalpel should be passed to the surgeon:

    a. Cutting edge pointing upward

    b. Cutting edge pointing downward

    c. In an emesis basin

    d. In two pieces and the surgeon will assemble it

24. Tissue forceps are passed to the surgeon:

    a. Pointed ends upward

    b. Cutting edge downward

    c. In position of function

    d. Immediately followed by scissors

25. Silk suture should not be pulled between gloved fingers. This prevents:

    a. Contamination of suture

    b. Formation of granuloma

    c. Breaks in suture

    d. Build-up of static electricity

26. When opening a package of absorbable suture, one opens the foil over a basin to:

    a. Prevent fluid from dripping on the table drape

    b. Prevent breakage of the suture

    c. Prevent cross-contamination

    d. Prevent build-up of static electricity

27. During passage of a tonsil with a tie in place, the tip should be:

    a. Pointed toward the scrub nurse

    b. Pointed toward the center of the surgeon's body

    c. Pointed downward and to the right

    d. Dipped in sterile water before being passed to the surgeon

28. Patient hypothermia is defined as a core temperature of:

    a. 34°C (93.2°F)

    b. 35°C (95°F)

    c. 36°C (96.8°F)

    d. 38°C (100.4°F)

29. The most effective method of reversing hypothermia is to:

    a. Maintain the procedure room air temperature at 26.7°C (80°F)

    b. Use convection air-warming devices

    c. Use hypothermia or hyperthermia water-filled mattresses

    d. Use warmed cotton blankets

30. Which of the following statements is true about convective warming therapy?

    a. An adverse effect of the convective warming therapy is the possibility of wound contamination secondary to an overly heated operative environment.

    b. Convective warming therapy is the most effective method of preventing or reversing hypothermia.

    c. Convective warming therapy transfers heat to the patient by blowing warm air through microperforations on the underside of a lightweight blanket that covers the patient.

d. Convective warming blankets are the recommended type of warming therapy for patients with compromised vascular perfusion.

31. When using a water-filled mattress during an operative or invasive procedure, the nurse will prevent the patient from receiving thermal burns or pressure necrosis by:

a. Checking the tubing and blanket for leaks

b. Preventing the patient's skin from coming into direct contact with the blanket

c. Checking the blanket for correct temperature by periodically placing a hand on the unit during the procedure

d. Ensuring that the blanket is flat without kinks or folds

32. Tourniquets are used to:

a. Decrease the need for local anesthesia

b. Decrease the length of operating time

c. Provide a bloodless field

d. Increase the patient's compliance

33. To ensure safe use of a pneumatic tourniquet, adequate gas is needed in the tank. How much pressure will be in the tank the perioperative nurse secures for the procedure?

a. 100 psi

b. 250 psi

c. 500 psi

d. 1000 psi

34. Tourniquet cuff size is important. The perioperative nurse will assess the patient and select a cuff that will overlap:

a. 1–3 inches

b. 3–6 inches

c. 6–10 inches

d. Not at all

35. Before inflating the tourniquet cuff, the surgeon will wrap the limb with Esmarch to:

a. Prevent the cuff from rotating during the procedure

b. Decrease the need for local anesthesia

c. Provide comfort to the patient

d. Compress veins and drain the blood from the limb

36. The nurse positions the tourniquet cuff:

a. Above the elbow or knee at the point of maximum circumference

b. Below the elbow or knee at the maximum circumference

c. At the elbow with equal distances above and below

d. At the brachial plexus

37. Excessive or insufficient tourniquet pressure may cause:

a. Necrosis of the skin

b. Nerve damage

c. Shearing of the skin

d. Blisters

38. The tourniquet cuff pressure for the arm of a healthy adult, to produce a bloodless field, should be:

a. 50–75 mm Hg above systolic pressure

b. 50–75 mm Hg above diastolic pressure

c. 100–150 mm Hg above systolic pressure

d. 100–150 mm Hg above diastolic pressure

39. An improper tourniquet cuff seal may result in:

a. Nerve damage

b. Bruising and blistering

c. Shearing of the skin

d. Burning

40. Seepage of preparation solution under the tourniquet cuff may result in:

a. Bruising

b. Nerve damage

c. Chemical burns

d. Shearing

41. Before applying the tourniquet cuff, the perioperative nurse applies:

a. Betadine solution

b. Vaseline

c. Bacitracin ointment

d. Wrinkle-free padding

42. As a general guideline, the tourniquet that is being used on an arm should be inflated for only:

a. 15 minutes

b. 30 minutes

c. 1 hour

d. 1 hour 30 minutes

43. All electrical equipment used on a patient should have a:

a. Grounded three-prong plug

b. Battery backup system

c. Nongrounded three-prong plug

d. Standby control mechanism

44. How will the nurse preserve the life of a battery and ensure enough energy to safely run the equipment?

a. Sterilize batteries in a hydrogen-peroxide sterilizer

b. Soak the instruments in a glutaraldehyde solution

c. Follow the manufacturer's written instructions

d. Use a new battery each time the equipment is used

45. What is the potential hazard when using an extension cord?

a. Macroshock

b. Alternate pathway burns

c. Insulation failure

d. Capacitive coupling

46. Electrosurgery should never be used when:

a. The patient has a pacemaker

b. A flammable anesthestic is being used

c. A pneumatic tourniquet is being used

d. The patient has a history of atrial fibrillation

47. Which of the following statements is true regarding electrosurgical general precautions?

a. Caution must be exercised when using electrosurgery during procedures in the thoracic cavity. A leak in lung tissue will produce a leak in methane gas, increasing the patient's risk for injury.

b. Many prepping solutions contain agents such as alcohol. Quick evaporation of these agents makes them safe to use with electrosurgery.

c. Electrosurgery is safe to use in the presence of hydrogen peroxide because hydrogen peroxide is an oxidizing agent that breaks down gas and produces oxygen.

d. Procedures in body cavities, particularly cavities in which gases can accumulate, pose a risk to the patient when using electrosurgery.

48. Electrosurgical units are not usually used with a patient with:

a. Metal prosthetic implants

b. Debilitating chronic diseases

c. Pacemakers

d. History of electrical burns

49. When using electrosurgery, the only time one would not use a patient return electrode would be when:

   a. The patient has an internal pacemaker

   b. Using bipolar accessories

   c. Regional anesthesia is used

   d. The patient has an allergy to the pad

50. What is the purpose of a patient return electrode during electrosurgery?

   a. It safely recovers the current that flows through the patient and returns it to the generator.

   b. It concentrates the current to prevent thermal burns to the patient.

   c. It limits the effect of the current to the tissue between the electrodes.

   d. It assists the electrical current to exit the patient's body at the smallest surface area.

51. What is the result of cutting a patient return electrode to reduce its size?

   a. The current will become concentrated and divert to the path of least resistance.

   b. The current will have difficulty exiting the patient.

   c. High current density will develop at the site of the cut.

   d. The generator will become disabled.

52. The nurse is about to apply a hydrogel adhesive electrode to the surgical patient. Before placing the pad, the nurse will:

   a. Lightly touch the surface of the hydrogel pad

   b. Attach the electrode cord to the generator

c. Clean the area with a degreaser

d. Inform the physician of his or her intentions

53. When should the patient return electrode be placed on the patient?

   a. Before induction of anesthesia

   b. After induction of anesthesia but before the surgical skin preparation

   c. After the patient is positioned

   d. After the surgical skin preparation

54. When placing the patient return electrode, why must one avoid areas of high impedance?

   a. These are areas of potential thermal burn.

   b. These are areas that would impede visibility to the surgical team.

   c. High-impedance areas may necessitate higher power settings.

   d. High-impedance areas may necessitate the use of a pacemaker.

55. The most likely place for burns due to alternate exit pathway of electrical current is at the:

   a. Pulse oximeter site

   b. Application site of electrocardiographic leads

   c. Hair line

   d. Base of the spine

56. The dispersive electrode should be placed:

   a. In a visible area

   b. At the farthest point from the incision site

   c. On the upper left arm

   d. Over a large muscle mass

57. The dispersive electrode should be removed when:

   a. The dressing has been applied and the drapes taken off

b. The incision has been closed

c. The counts are completed

d. The patient arrives in the post-anesthesia care unit

58. If the active electrode and return patient electrode cords are coiled or bundled, there is potential for:

a. Electrical leakage

b. Current concentration

c. Cardiac arrhythmias

d. Electrocardiographic artifact

59. A cast should be removed outside the restricted areas of the surgical suite to:

a. Decrease the cost of the procedure

b. Prevent cross-contamination

c. Guarantee patient privacy

d. Confine the plaster dust

60. To slow plaster setting time, the physician will:

a. Remove excess water from the plaster roll

b. Add salt to the water

c. Add calcium gluconate to the water

d. Leave excessive amounts of water in the plaster roll

61. If the surgeon applies the tape to the sterile dressing, he or she should remove the gloves to:

a. Stretch the skin smoothly

b. Prevent cross-contamination

c. Facilitate drape removal

d. Speed the procedure along

62. Plaster of Paris is made from:

a. Calcium gluconate

b. Sulfur

c. Hydrous calcium sulfate

d. Cotton

63. Plaster setting times can be accelerated by:

a. Removing excess water from the plaster roll

b. Adding cold water to water already in the bucket

c. Leaving excessive amounts of water in plaster rolls

d. Adding sugar to water in the bucket

64. Padding the cast reduces the risk of:

a. Chemical burns

b. Hypothermia

c. Pressure sore formation

d. Nerve damage

65. To prevent cast denting, the cast is:

a. Covered with stockinet

b. Protected from contacting rough surfaces

c. Painted with a solution of sugar and normal saline

d. Molded until the plaster is shiny

66. When dipping a plaster roll, it is held in a vertical position to:

a. Force water out of the roll

b. Create a smooth surface

c. Prevent splashing water around sterile field

d. Allow air to escape through the core of the roll

67. Most casts are removed:

a. With hydrogen peroxide and a plaster knife

b. By soaking it in a bucket of warm water

c. With an electrical cast cutter

d. By creating grooves, then pouring gentian violet into those grooves

68. The tape is applied to the sterile dressing by the:

a. Circulating nurse

b. Scrub nurse

c. Surgeon

d. Anesthesia personnel

69. Who is responsible for maintaining the endoscopic video equipment?

a. Circulating nurse

b. Scrub person

c. Biomedical engineering department

d. Physician

70. To allow visualization during laparoscopy, the abdomen is distended with:

a. Ambient air

b. Sterile water

c. Carbon dioxide

d. Ether

71. Which statement is true regarding laparoscopic insufflation?

a. Carbon dioxide is instilled because it will not form a gas embolus.

b. The carbon dioxide supply bottle should be at a 45-degree angle when in use.

c. Risks associated with the establishment of a pneumoperitoneum depend on physician skill.

d. Perforation of an abdominal vessel is the only risk that would necessitate an open laparotomy.

■ Answers

1. [a] Extended anesthesia time

Without organization or protocols in place, the simple task of selecting instruments, equipment, supplies, and sutures for an operative or invasive procedure becomes complicated and may adversely affect patient outcomes. The primary concern is an extended anesthesia time, which may have adverse cardiac, respiratory, neurological, or integumentary effects on the patient. (*page 97*)

2. [d] Compromise of the package compromises sterility.

The shelf life of a packaged sterile item is event related. Compromise of the package compromises sterility. The item should not be used if a defect in packaging is found. (*page 97*)

3. [d] Type of anesthesia, cold room, and decreased body fat

Risk factors associated with altered body temperature during surgery include general or regional anesthesia, use of unwarmed fluids, extremes in age, decreased body fat, chronic illness, preexisting medical conditions (hypothyroid or hyperthyroid problems), and a cold room. (*page 99*)

4. [c] Open the item on a separate table

Sharp, bulky, or heavy objects should be presented to the scrub person or opened on a separate surface, such as a table or Mayo stand. (*page 98*)

5. [d] Discard the unused portion of solution

The edge of the container is considered contaminated after the cap has been removed. Therefore, unused fluids are discarded. (*page 98*)

6. [c] Close towel clip box locks

Towel clip box locks are closed to prevent accidental puncture of sterile gloves, and they are returned to the rolled towel. (*page 98*)

7. [a] Alterations in temperature or electrical injury

Outcome standard: *The patient is free from injury related to provision of instruments, equipment, and supplies during the surgery will be demonstrated by no alteration in temperature, electrical injury, burns, or nosocomial infections.* (*page 98*)

8. [c] Excessive hair, pacemaker

Risk factors associated with high risk for injury related to the use of electrical equipment include: excessive hair at patient return electrode site, scar tissue at patient return electrode site, internal/external metal prosthetic devices, pacemakers, bony prominence at patient return electrode site, obesity, emaciation. (*page 100*)

9. [c] High risk for infection

Risk factors associated with Nosocomial Infection include: failure of sterilization or disinfection process, nonadherence to aseptic technique, failure of environmental sanitation, nutritional status of the patient, medications (steroids, chemotherapy), high white blood counts, and compromise of the immune system. (*page 99*)

10. [b] Inadequate secondary defenses

Risk factors associated with high risk for infection include: inadequate secondary defenses, inadequate acquired immunity, chronic disease, malnutrition, impaired skin integrity, impaired tissue integrity. (*page 99*)

11. [a] Chemical burns or nerve damage

The patient is free from injury related to pneumatic tourniquet use, there is no evidence of bruising, blisters, skin abrasions or swelling, chemical burns, paralysis, or signs of nerve damage. (*page 99*)

12. [b] Alteration in tissue perfusion

The patient is free from electrical equipment-related injury evidenced by no impaired skin and tissue integrity, altered tissue perfusion, altered cardiac output, or impaired neurological function. (*page 100*)

13. [a] *Patient's body temperature maintained within normal limits*

Expected outcome for high risk for altered body temperature during surgery: *Patient's body temperature is maintained within normal limits evidenced by no shivering, chattering of teeth, or cool skin.* (*page 99*)

14. [d] Injury related to use of pneumatic tourniquet

Risk factors associated with high risk for injury related to use of pneumatic tourniquet are improper cuff size, wrinkled padding, pooling of preparation solution under the cuff, and excessive cuff pressure. (*page 99*)

15. [b] Hypothyroidism

Risk factors associated with hypothermia include cold operating room, general and regional anesthesia, cool skin preparations, preexisting medical conditions (hypothyroidism or hyperthyroidism) extremes in ages, malnourishment, intracranial procedures, and hypovolemia. (*page 99*)

16. [a] Injury related to extended anesthesia time

Risk factors associated with risk for injury related to extended anesthesia time include inaccurate and outdated physician preference cards, inadequate inventory of necessary supplies and implants, equipment not procured or checked for function before induction of anesthesia, and instruments not reprocessed and sterilized in a timely manner. (*page 99*)

17. [c] Patient is free from injury related to pneumatic tourniquet use

When the patient is free from injury related to the use of a pneumatic tourniquet, there is no evidence of bruising, blisters, pinching, or necrosis of skin. (*page 99*)

18. [a] Away from the body

The autoclave tape on the wrapped item is broken by the opener. The package is opened by first lifting the top flap away from the body. The second and third flaps are lifted to the right and left, and the last flap is lifted toward the opener. (*page 97*)

19. [b] Flip items onto sterile field

If the scrub nurse cannot accept the sterile item, the circulating nurse should flip the item onto the sterile field. If the item touches the inner seal while being passed to the sterile field, it is considered contaminated. (*page 98*)

20. [d] It has been dropped on the floor

Do not use cloth- or paper-wrapped items that are dropped on the floor. If a package defect is found, the item is considered contaminated. (*page 97*)

21. [a] Needle holder

The scalpel blade is loaded on the handle by holding the scalpel handle in one's non-dominant hand. The dominant hand grasps the blade on the dull edge with a needle holder at the widest, strongest point without touching the cutting edge. The blade and handle are pointed down and away from the body, and the blade is slid into the groove of the scalpel handle until it is secure. (*page 100*)

22. [d] Uniformly set up

To facilitate continuity of care during the staff changes in the operating room, all specialties should have standard back table and Mayo tray setups. (*page 98*)

23. [c] In an emesis basin

To prevent injuries, the hands-free technique is used when passing the scalpel, needle, or other sharp instruments. When using this technique, one lays the secured needle or sharp item down in a designated neutral zone on the sterile field. (*page 101*)

24. [c] In position of function

Tissue forceps and ringed or box-locked instruments are passed in position of function. Multipiece retractors should be assembled before they are passed to the physician or assistant. Retractors are passed handle first. (*page 101*)

25. [d] Build-up of static electricity

Avoiding pulling silk suture between gloved fingers prevents build-up of static electricity in the suture. The strands are placed under the towel on the Mayo tray according to type and size. (*page 101*)

26. [a] Prevent fluid from dripping on the table drape

The foil package should be carefully torn over a small basin to prevent fluid from dripping on the table drape. (*page 101*)

27. [b] Pointed toward the center of the surgeon's body

The tip of the suture strand is placed securely into the tip of a tonsil clamp or a right angle clamp, and the clamp is locked. The clamp should be gently slapped into the palm of the surgeon's hand with the tip of the clamp pointing toward the center of the surgeon's body. (*page 101*)

28. [c] 36°C (96.8°F)

Patient hypothermia is defined as a core temperature of 36.8°C (96.8°F). (*page 101*)

29. [a] Maintain the procedure room air temperature at 26.7°C (80°F)

The most effective method of preventing or reversing hypothermia is to maintain the procedure room air temperture at 26.7°C—29.4°C (80°–85°F). These temperatures are too warm for team members dressed in full scrub attire and working under spotlights. (*page 101*)

30. [c] Convective warming therapy transfers heat to the patient by blowing warm air through microperforations on the underside of a lightweight blanket that covers the patient.

Convective warming therapy has been found to be more effective than the water-filled warming mattress or other commonly suggested methods of patient warming. Convective warming therapy transfers heat to the patient by blowing warm air through microperforations on the underside of a lightweight blanket that covers the patient. (*page 101*)

31. [b] Preventing the patient's skin from coming into direct contact with the blanket

Thermal burns or pressure necrosis may occur with a hyperthermia or hypothermia blanket. Therefore, unless the blanket is designed for direct contact, the blanket should be covered with an absorbable pad or sheet. (*page 102*)

32. [c] Provide a bloodless field

Tourniquets are used to provide a bloodless field. Pneumatic tourniquet equipment includes a pressure source, a pressure gauge, a regulator, tubing, connectors, and an inflatable cuff. (*page 102*)

33. [c] 500 psi

The pressure source must be checked for adequate gas. An inert nonflammable gas, such as nitrogen or room air, is used to inflate the cuff. Pressure in the tank should read at least 500 psi. (*page 102*)

34. [b] 3–6 inches

Use of inappropriate-sized cuffs can injure the patient. The patient should be assessed for extremity size and a cuff selected that overlaps at the ends by 3–6 inches. (*page 102*)

35. [d] Compress veins and drain the blood from the limb

The surgeon may wrap the extremity tightly with a 4–6-inch Esmarch or elastic bandage before inflating the cuff to compress the veins and drain blood from the limb. (*page 102*)

36. [a] Above the elbow or knee at the point of maximum circumference

The nurse positions the tourniquet cuff on the limb at the most proximal point of maximum circumference, according to the manufacturer's written instructions. (*page 102*)

37. [b] Nerve damage

The pressure gauge must be clearly visible and the cuff monitored periodically during inflation for pressure fluctuations. Excessive or insufficient tourniquet pressure can cause nerve damage. (*page 102*)

38. [a] 50–75 mm Hg above systolic pressure

As a guideline, in healthy adult patients, 50–75 mm Hg above systolic pressure for arms and 100–150 mm Hg above systolic pressure for legs usually produces a bloodless field. Pressures are lower for children and patients with impaired perfusion. Tourniquet pressure should impede arterial blood flow, not venous flow. (*page 102*)

39. [b] Bruising and blistering

An incomplete or overly aggressive seal of the cuff must be avoided. An improper cuff seal can result in bruising, blistering, pinching, or necrosis of the skin. (*page 102*)

40. [c] Chemical burns

Pooling of antimicrobial solutions with the subsequent pressure of the inflated cuff may result in chemical burns. If preparation solutions seep under the cuff, the cuff must be removed and a moist cloth used to wipe the prepping solution from the extremity. The extremity is then dried and the cuff reapplied. (*page 102*)

41. [d] Wrinkle-free padding

Before applying the tourniquet, the nurse applies wrinkle-free padding unless contraindicated by the manufacturer. When applied correctly, the padding protects the skin under the cuff from mechanical injury. (*page 102*)

42. [c] 1 hour

Exact tourniquet times have not been established. As a general guideline, the tourniquet should stay inflated no longer than 1 hour. (*page 103*)

43. [a] Grounded three-prong plug

All electrical equipment used on a patient should have a grounded three-prong plug. Nongrounded equipment could potentially provide enough current leakage to cause microshock in a cardiac-compromised patient. (*page 103*)

44. [c] Follow the manufacturer's written instructions

To preserve the life of batteries and ensure enough energy to safely run the equipment, the manufacturer's written instructions for charging and sterilizing the batteries must be followed. (*page 104*)

45. [a] Macroshock

Use of extension cords may result in macroshock or microshock. (*page 104*)

46. [b] A flammable anesthestic is being used

Electrosurgery is never used in the presence of flammable anesthetics or other flammable gases, flammable liquids, or flammable objects. (*page 104*)

47. [d] Procedures in body cavities, particularly cavities in which gases can accumulate, pose a risk to the patient when using electrosurgery.

Procedures in body cavities, particularly cavities in which gases can accumulate, pose a risk to the patient. During abdominal procedures, especially procedures in which naturally occurring gases such as methane gas may be present, electrosurgery must be used with caution. (*page 104*)

48. [c] Pacemakers

If the patient has an external or internal pacemaker, electrosurgery must be used with extreme caution. The electrosurgery generator can cause pacemakers to enter an asynchronous mode or can completely block the effect of the pacemaker. (*page 104*)

49. [b] Using bipolar accessories

A patient return electrode is not necessary for a bipolar procedure when only bipolar accessories are used. If a patient return electrode is used, the electrosurgical effect may not be limited to the tissue between the bipolar electrodes. (*page 105*)

50. [a] It safely recovers the current that flows through the patient and returns it to the generator.

During monopolar electrosurgery, a patient return electrode should always be applied to the patient. The patient return electrode safely recovers the current that flows through the patient and returns it to the generator. (*page 105*)

51. [c] High current density will develop at the site of the cut.

If the patient return electrode is too large, cutting the electrode to reduce its size is not an option. Cutting the patient return electrode causes high current density at the site of the cut and may burn the patient. (*page 106*)

52. [a] Lightly touch the surface of the hydrogel pad

Before applying a hydrogel adhesive electrode, the nurse lightly touches the surface of the hydrogel to ensure that the conductive adhesive is moist. The electrode is discarded if the adhesive is not moist. (*page 106*)

53. [c] After the patient is positioned

The patient return electrode is placed after the patient is in position. The electrode is attached to a clean, dry skin surface, over a wall-vascularized, large muscle mass, and in a convex area close to the procedure site. (*page 106*)

54. [c] High-impedence areas may necessitate the use of higher power settings

High-impedence areas to be avoided include bony prominences, scar tissue, skin over an implanted metal prosthesis, hairy surfaces, pressure points, and adipose tissue. Placing a patient return electrode over a high impedence area may necessitate higher power settings. (*page 106*)

55. [b] Application site of electrocardiographic leads

The most likely place for burns due to alternate exit pathways of electrical current is the application site for electrocardiographic leads. (*page 105*)

56. [d] Over a large muscle mass

The dispersive electrode pad should be placed over a large muscle mass close to the incision site, not over bony prominences, scar tissue, areas with large metal prosthetic implants, or excessively hairy areas. (*page 106*)

57. [a] The dressing has been applied and the drapes taken off

After the dressing has been applied and the drapes have been removed from the patient, the patient return electrode is carefully peeled from the patient's skin. The patient is evaluated using the expected outcome criteria identified for *Risk for Injury related to electrosurgery*. (*page 107*)

58. [b] Current concentration

Active electrode and return patient electrode cords must not be coiled or bundled. Coiling and bundling cause current concentration and create a fire hazard as well as a potential burn site for the patient. (*page 108*)

59. [d] Confine the plaster dust

An electric cast cutter with an attached vacuum is used to remove a cast. The cast should be removed outside the restricted area of the surgical suite to confine plaster dust. The patient should be reassured that he or she will not be cut as the cast is removed. (*page 109*)

60. [d] Leave excessive amounts of water in the plaster roll

Plaster setting time can be slowed by leaving excessive amounts of water in the plaster roll or by immersing the roll in cool water. (*page 108*)

61. [b] Prevent cross-contamination

The surgeon should remove his or her gloves to prevent cross-contamination when applying tape. (*page 108*)

62. [c] Hydrous calcium sulfate

Plaster of Paris is made from hydrous calcium sulfate. Setting times are deter-

mined by chemicals added to the plaster. (*page 108*)

63. [a] Removing excess water from the plaster roll

The physician may accelerate the set time by removing excess water from the plaster roll, by rubbing and working with the plaster as it is applied, or by immersing the roll in warmer water. (*page 108*)

64. [c] Pressure sore formation

The physician applies padding smoothly over the stockinet, in one to three layers, with turns overlapping about half the width of the bandage. Pieces of heavy felt can be placed over bony prominences to reduce the risk of skin breakdown. (*page 108*)

65. [b] Protected from contacting rough surfaces

To prevent cast denting, the extremity is elevated on a pillow and the cast is protected from contacting rough surfaces. (*page 109*)

66. [d] Allow air to escape through the core of the roll

The plaster roll is held in a vertical position to allow air to escape through the core of the roll as it is dipped in the water. (*page 108*)

67. [c] With an electrical cast cutter

Most casts are removed with an electrical cast cutter with a vacuum attached to keep the dust confined. (*page 109*)

68. [a] Circulating nurse

The circulating nurse secures the dressing with tape. The skin must not be stretched while the tape is applied. (*page 108*)

69. [a] Circulating nurse

The circulating nurse is responsible for ensuring that the equipment is functioning correctly and that he or she has an accurate visual image. This requires a thorough knowledge of the manufacturer's operating instructions and the interface of the system components. (*page 109*)

70. [c] Carbon dioxide

During laparoscopy, the abdomen is distended with medical-grade carbon dioxide instilled through a Veres needle inserted into the peritoneal cavity through a small para-umbilical incision, thereby allowing the physician to visualize, manipulate, and operate on the abdominal organs. (*page 110*)

71. [c] Risks associated with the establishment of a pneumoperitoneum depend on physician skill.

There are risks associated with the establishment of a pneumoperitoneum. The risks depend on physician skill, the type of gas used to produce the pneumoperitonium, the level of intra-abdominal pressure, and the functioning of instruments during the procedure. (*page 110*)

CHAPTER **8**

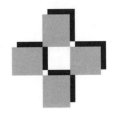

Administering Drugs and Solutions

The nurse must ensure that drugs or solutions are administered to the patient according to hospital policy, manufacturers' recommendations, applicable federal and state regulations and laws, and recommended nursing practices. Before administering drugs and solutions, the nurse identifies the patient's risk for adverse outcomes related to the administration of drugs and solutions, the nursing diagnoses that describe the degrees of risk, and expected patient outcomes. After the identification of risks, diagnoses, and outcomes, the nurse plans interventions for care. After administering drugs and solutions, the nurse evaluates the effectiveness of interventions according to criteria delineated in the expected outcome. The questions for this chapter will help the reader assess his or her knowledge about

- Recognizing potential adverse drugs and solution reaction
- Describing the pharmacological characteristics of drugs and solutions used during operative and invasive procedures
- Describing the human response to the administration of drugs and solutions
- Obtaining a medical history
- Identifying patients at risk for adverse outcomes related to the administration of drugs and solutions
- Gathering supplies and equipment
- Preparing and administering drugs and solutions according to institutional policy, manufacturers' recommendations, federal and state regulations, and recommended nursing practice

The reference used for this chapter is Phippen, M. L., & Wells, M. P. (1999). *Patient care during operative and invasive procedures.* Philadelphia: W. B. Saunders, pp. 113–135.

✚ Questions

1. During a surgical procedure, preparing and administering drugs and solutions is a shared responsibility between:

   a. The circulating nurse and scrub nurse

   b. The circulating nurse and surgeon

   c. The circulating nurse, first assistant, scrub person, and surgeon

   d. The surgeon and first assistant

2. During a surgical procedure, the circulating nurse receives an oral order from the surgeon to prepare an irrigation solution of bacitracin and normal saline. What actions should be taken after the order is given to the circulating nurse?

   a. After preparing the solution, the circulating nurse places it on the operative field. The scrub person labels the solution and identifies it each time it is administered.

   b. The circulating nurse verifies this order with the surgeon, prepares the solution, and places it on the operative field. The scrub person labels the solution and identifies it each time it is administered.

   c. The circulating nurse verifies this order with the surgeon, prepares the solution, and places it on the operative field. The scrub person identifies it each time it is administered.

   d. The circulating nurse verifies this order with the surgeon, prepares the solution, and places it on the operative field. The scrub person labels the solution.

3. Toxicity is usually caused by:

   a. Drug allergy

   b. Drug hypersensitivity

   c. Improper mixing of drugs

   d. Drug overdose

4. Drug allergy and idiosyncrasy are the result of a patient's sensitivity to:

   a. A drug's secondary pharmacological effects

   b. A specific chemical

   c. A specific preservative

   d. A drug's primary pharmacological effects

5. A reaction due to drug allergy occurs:

   a. Only after the individual becomes sensitized

   b. At the first administration

   c. At the second administration

   d. Within minutes after exposure

6. If a patient has an anaphylactic reaction to a drug, signs and symptoms develop within minutes after exposure. Which of the following statements are true?

   (1) These reactions result from the release of active chemical mediators during the antibody reactions.

   (2) The degree of severity depends on how much of the drug was administered.

   (3) These reactions result from the release of active chemical mediators during the antigen-antibody reactions.

   (4) The degree of severity does not depend on the drug but on how strongly sensitized the individual was when she or he received the drug at an earlier time.

   a. (1) and (4)

   b. (2) and (3)

   c. (1) and (3)

   d. (3) and (4)

7. In a delayed drug reaction, the appearance of signs and symptoms may not be evident until several hours or days after exposure to the chemical. Signs and symptoms of a delayed reaction may include:

   a. Contact dermatitis and hemolytic anemia, fever, swollen lymph nodes, and edema of the face and limbs

   b. Abdominal cramping, diarrhea, contact dermatitis and hemolytic anemia, fever, swollen lymph nodes, and edema of the face and limbs

   c. Abdominal cramping, diarrhea, fever, swollen lymph nodes, and edema of the face and limbs

   d. Severe urticaria, diarrhea, fever, swollen lymph nodes, and generalized edema

8. Patients who are abnormally sensitive to small doses of a drug the first time it is administered may experience:

   a. A hypersensitivity reaction

   b. An allergic reaction

   c. A toxic reaction

   d. An idiosyncratic reaction

9. In a low-weight patient, the reactive target tissue receives a greater portion of the dose. Consequently, the effect of the drug on the low-weight patient is:

   a. Lesser than that on a heavier patient

   b. Greater than that on a heavier patient

   c. The same as that on a heavier patient

   d. Minimal

10. Inadequate primary defense, inadequate secondary defense, malnutrition, and extremes of age are risk factors associated with what nursing diagnosis?

   a. *Risk for Fluid Volume Deficit related to the use of heparin*

b. *Risk for Infection related to the administration of drugs and solutions*

c. *Risk for Injury related to hypersensitivity or an adverse reaction to an antiplatelet agent*

d. *Risk for Injury related to toxicity from local anesthetic*

11. Mrs. Smith is scheduled for a mitral valve replacement. She is 72 years old and has a history of diverticulitis. The operative and invasive procedure nurse recognizes that Mrs. Smith may be at risk for:

    a. Injury related to an allergic reaction to local anesthesia

    b. Infection related to the administration of drugs and solutions

    c. Fluid volume deficit (blood loss) related to the use of heparin

    d. Injury related to toxicity from local anesthetic

12. Which of the following statements is true regarding the risk factors associated with the nursing diagnosis *Risk for Injury related to hypersensitivity or an adverse reaction to an anticoagulant or antiplatelet agent*?

    a. Mrs. Walter is a 49-year-old woman about to have an emergency surgical procedure because of a motor vehicle accident. There are no family members present, and Mrs. Walter is disoriented and unable to provide a medical history.

    b. Mrs. Walter has a history of six surgical procedures to repair a ruptured femoral aneurysm.

    c. Mrs. Walter had a severe reaction to Profenol during a previous surgical procedure.

    d. Mrs. Walter is known to metabolize lidocaine slowly.

13. Hospital policy dictates that patient weight be recorded in kilograms. During the preoperative assessment, the nurse notes that the patient weighs 185 lb. The nurse should record this weight as:

    a. 86 kg

    b. 120 kg

    c. 84 kg

    d. 100 kg

14. During the cataract procedure, the physician asks for epinephrine to be added to the irrigating solution. Ten minutes after the drug is added, the nurse notices that Mr. James' electrocardiogram (ECG) is showing increased numbers of premature ventricular contractions. This is a risk factor associated with which nursing diagnosis:

    a. *Risk associated with allergic reaction to contrast media*

    b. *Risk of Fluid Volume Deficit related to the administration of hyperosmotic agents*

    c. *Risk for Decreased Cardiac Output related to toxicity from a local anesthetic*

    d. *Risk for Injury related to administration of mydriatic agents*

15. Why would diabetes place a patient at risk for fluid volume deficit related to the administration of hyperosmotic agents?

    a. Osmotic agents can cause hyperglycemia and glycosuria.

    b. Osmotic agents precipitate dehydration in diabetic patients.

    c. Diabetic patients are more sensitive to increases in fluid volume.

    d. Diabetic patients have a history of renal dysfunction.

16. Mrs. Chan is scheduled for a cholecystectomy with possible cholangiogram. She has a history of bronchial asthma and hay fever. She states that she has trouble

breathing when she eats shellfish. What nursing diagnosis most fits Mrs. Chan?

a. *Risk for Injury related to mydriatic agent administration*

b. *Risk for Injury related to an allergic reaction to contrast media*

c. *Risk for Fluid Volume Deficit related to the administration of hyperosmotic agents*

d. *Risk for Fluid Volume Excess related to the absorption of large amounts of endoscopic irrigating fluid into the systemic circulation*

17. Existing disease states can alter drug metabolism and excretion and cause an unexpected drug response. Which statement is true?

a. A patient with severe liver disease is a poor candidate for general anesthesia with Halothane (Fluothane) because the final elimination of this drug from the body requires enzymatic breakdown in the liver.

b. A patient with severe liver disease is a poor candidate for local anesthesia with lidocaine hydrochloride (Xylocaine) because the final elimination of this drug from the body requires enzymatic breakdown in the liver.

c. A patient with severe liver disease is a poor candidate for general anesthesia with Propofol (Diprivan) because the final elimination of this drug from the body requires enzymatic breakdown in the liver.

d. A patient with severe renal dysfunction is a poor candidate for general anesthesia with halothane (Fluothane) because the final elimination of this drug from the body requires enzymatic breakdown in the liver.

18. When does cross-tolerance to a drug develop?

a. The patient continues to take a drug for a long period of time.

b. The drug is ingested at a greater rate than the rate at which it can be eliminated.

c. Different drugs are taken that act at the same cellular level to produce similar effects.

d. The patient has severe medical limitations for drug metabolism, such as diabetes, cancer, or cardiovascular disease.

19. The effect produced when drugs are ingested at a greater rate than the rate at which they can be eliminated is known as:

a. Cumulative effect

b. Cross-tolerance

c. Drug tolerance

d. Inhibited effect

20. An inborn ability to remain unaffected by certain anti-infective drugs is:

a. Active immunity

b. Passive immunity

c. Microbial resistance

d. Congenital resistance

21. A bactericidal agent will:

a. Have a direct action on the bacteria that will result in destruction or death of the bacteria

b. Inhibit the growth of the bacteria

c. Prevent an allergic reaction to the microorganism

d. Identify various types of bacteria

22. Protection against a pathogen and its toxins by transfer of antibodies produced in the body of another individual or animal that has been actively immunized is known as:

a. Active immunity

b. Passive immunity

c. Congenital immunity

d. Microbial immunity

23. Psychological factors influence a patient's willingness to take a medication. Which of the following statements is also true?

a. The degree of drug effectiveness *is never* affected by psychological factors.

b. The degree of drug effectiveness *may be* affected by psychological factors.

c. The degree of drug effectiveness *may be* affected by psychological factors *depending* on the amount of drug administered.

d. The degree of drug effectiveness *is always* affected by psychological factors.

24. During the preoperative assessment the nurse assesses the patient's value-belief pattern to:

a. Determine whether the patient believes in a deity

b. Determine the patient's willingness to submit to the administration of investigational drugs

c. Determine whether the patient has religious beliefs that may influence medication administration and compliance

d. Determine whether certain medications are contraindicated because of the patient's religious beliefs

25. The first attempt by the federal government to prevent drug abuse in the medical and nursing communities occurred in 1914. This legislation was called the:

a. Drug Abuse Amendments

b. Durham-Humphrey Amendment

c. Comprehensive Drug Abuse Prevention and Control Act

d. Harrison Narcotic Act

26. Emergency treatment of infections before the causative agent is known is often begun with a combination of how many broad-spectrum drugs?

a. Two

b. One

c. Three

d. Four

27. A serious form of anti-infective agent related toxicity may:

a. Occur following intravenous administration

b. Occur when absorbed antibiotics are poorly eliminated and accumulate in the tissue

c. Result in phlebitis

d. Result in anaphylactic shock

28. Allergies have been reported with almost every kind of anti-infective drug. Reactions are most common with:

a. Aminoglycosides

b. Cephalosporin

c. Penicillin

d. Tetracycline

29. The goal of preoperative and intraoperative chemoprophylaxis is to:

a. Destroy microorganisms

b. Prevent implantation and invasion by a specific pathogen

c. Prevent wound infection

d. Prevent a systemic infection

30. Prostheses, such as penile, testicular, breast, and orthopedic implants, are commonly soaked in an antibiotic solution before being implanted. Commonly used antibiotics include:

a. Bacitracin, polymyxin B, and gentamicin

b. Bacitracin, garamycin, and nystatin

c. Bacitracin, garamycin, and gentamicin

d. Bacitracin, polymyxin B, and doxycycline

31. This drug is often administered before surgery to reduce the incidence of postoperative infections in patients undergoing surgical procedures classified as contaminated or potentially contaminated. It is also given when infections at the operative site present risk (e.g., for prosthetic arthroplasty and cardiothoracic and vascular procedures). What is it?

a. Garamycin

b. Tetracycline

c. Cefonicid sodium

d. Penicillin G

32. The phase of homeostasis that prevents propagation of clotting beyond the site of injury is the:

a. First

b. Second

c. Third

d. Fourth

33. What is the purpose of administering anticoagulants?

a. Prevent the extension of clots

b. Dissolve existing clots

c. Cause platelets to aggregate at the cell wall

d. Speed the natural clot-resolving process

34. The drug that acts in the liver to prevent the synthesis of vitamin K–dependent clotting factors and prevents coagulation is:

a. Heparin

b. Warfarin

c. Dextran 40

d. Dipyridamole

35. Before administering dextran 40, the nurse should check the chart for what?

a. Liver function studies

b. Hematocrit

c. Prothrombin time

d. History of food allergy

36. A solid mass of clotted blood in a vessel or in the heart is known as:

a. Hematoma

b. Petechia

c. Thrombus

d. Embolus

37. What is a hematoma?

a. A small spot caused by bleeding in the skin or mucous membranes

b. A localized collection of blood in a space, organ, or tissue

c. A solid mass of clotted blood in the heart

d. A clot carried by the blood from a larger vessel to a smaller vessel

38. Why is epinephrine added to local anesthetic solutions?

a. To interrupt the conduction of nerve impulses

b. To speed up the absorption of the local anesthetic agent

c. To slow down the absorption of the local anesthetic agent

d. To cause vasodilation

39. A block that affects the roots of nerves at various points close to their origin in the spinal cord is known as a:

a. Field block

b. Peripheral nerve block

c. Intravenous nerve block

d. Central nerve block

40. The perioperative nurse is preparing an epinephrine solution. The nurse is using 50 mL of normal saline. To have a final concentration of 1:200,000, how much epinephrine (1:1000 mL) will be added?

a. 0.25 mL

b. 0.30 mL

c. 0.40 mL

d. 0.50 mL

41. When are cycloplegic agents contraindicated?

a. The patient has glaucoma.

b. The patient will be under general anesthesia.

c. The patient is allergic to shellfish.

d. The patient has a history of hypertension.

42. When instilling eyedrops, what can the nurse do to lessen systemic absorption of the drug?

a. Administer eyedrops 1 hour before the operative procedure.

b. Apply pressure to the inner canthus.

c. Have the patient tightly close the eyelids immediately.

d. Warm the medication before instilling the drops.

43. Medications that directly cause the sphincter muscles of the iris to contract are known as:

a. Adrenergic agents

b. Cholinergic agents

c. Miotic agents

d. Mydriatric agents

44. What are miotic agents primarily used for?

a. Cataract surgery

b. Enhance the effects of anesthetic agents

c. Glaucoma

d. Irrigating solution

45. Which of the following drugs would be contraindicated for a patient with herpes simplex?

a. Glycerin

b. Hyaluronidase

c. Hyaluronate sodium (Healon)

d. Hydrocortisone

46. Which of the following statements describes a type III drug allergy?

a. Anaphylaxis or an acute reaction that results in cardiovascular/respiratory collapse

b. Occurs when the foreign antigen adheres to the surface of the host's cells; antibodies are then formed by the host, which attack the target cells

c. Anaphylatoxins and neutrophils release necrotizing enzymes that produce local ischemia and necrosis as a consequence of complement activation

d. A cell-mediated hypersensitivity reaction that is mediated through T lymphocytes rather than antibodies

47. The patient position of choice during eyedrop instillation would be:

a. Supine

b. Semilateral

c. Standing

d. Prone

48. How can the patient reduce the blinking reflex during installation of ophthalmic ointment?

a. Look upward

b. Look downward

c. Apply pressure to the inner canthus

d. Apply pressure to the nasolacrimal duct

49. For what condition would protamine sulfate be contraindicated?

   a. Glaucoma

   b. Allergy to seafood

   c. Hypertension

   d. Never

50. Which of the following statements is true about endoscopic procedures?

   a. When warming solutions for endoscopic procedures, it is important to remember to heat the container to 75°C.

   b. The container should be elevated at least 90 cm above the procedure bed.

   c. Most adverse reactions from endoscopic procedures do not occur until 24 hours after the procedure.

   d. Excessive elevation of the container can increase intravascular absorption of the irrigating fluid.

✚ Answers

1. [c] The circulating nurse, first assistant, scrub person, and surgeon

During a surgical procedure, the circulating nurse, first assistant, scrub person, and surgeon share in the responsibility for preparing and administering drugs and solutions during the intraoperative phase. Each team member is responsible for patient safety as it relates to identifying the patient and verifying the name of the medication, the dosage, the administration route, and the time and frequency of administration. (*page 113*)

2. [b] The circulating nurse verifies the order with the surgeon, prepares the

solution, and places it on the operative field. The scrub person labels the solution and identifies it each time it is administered.

During a surgical procedure, the circulating nurse receives an oral order from the surgeon to prepare an irrigation solution of bacitracin and normal saline. After receiving the order, the circulating nurse verifies this order with the surgeon, prepares the solution, places it on the operative field. The scrub person labels the solution and identifies it each time it is administered. (*page 113*)

3. [d] Drug overdose

Toxicity is usually caused by drug overdose. When this occurs, it is an adverse effect of the drug's known pharmacological characteristics. If the dose is large enough, toxic effects can occur in any patient. Even with small doses, toxicity is possible if the patient is hypersusceptible to one or another of the drug's primary or secondary pharmacological effects. (*page 114*)

4. [b] A specific chemical

Drug allergy and idiosyncrasy are the result of a patient's sensitivity to a specific chemical. These conditions differ from toxicity in that they are not related to the drug's pharmacology. (*page 114*)

5. [a] Only after the individual becomes sensitized

Drug allergy and idiosyncrasy result because of a patient's sensitivity to a specific chemical. A reaction due to drug allergy does not occur at the first time of administration but only after the individual becomes sensitized. (*page 114*)

6. [d] (3) and (4)

If a patient has an anaphylactic reaction to a drug, signs and symptoms develop within minutes after exposure. These reactions result from the release of active chemical mediators during the antigen-antibody reactions. The degree of severity does not depend on the drug but on how strongly sensitized the individual was when she or he received the drug at an earlier time. (*page 114*)

7. [a] Contact dermatitis and hemolytic anemia, fever, swollen lymph nodes, and edema of the face and limbs

In a delayed drug reaction, the appearance of signs and symptoms may not be evident until several hours or days after exposure to the chemical. Signs and symptoms of a delayed reaction may include contact dermatitis and hemolytic anemia, fever, swollen lymph nodes, and edema of the face and limbs. (*page 114*)

8. [d] An idiosyncratic reaction

Patients who are abnormally sensitive to small doses of a drug the first time it is administered may experience an idiosyncratic reaction. Malignant hyperthermia is an example. This uncommon response may occur in patients who receive inhalation anesthetics such as halothane or the skeletal muscle relaxant succinylcholine. (*page 114*)

9. [b] Greater than that on a heavier patient

In a low-weight patient, the reactive target tissue receives a greater portion of the dose. Consequently, the effect of the drug on a low-weight patient is greater than that on a heavier patient. (*page 114*)

10. [b] *Risk for Infection related to the administration of drugs and solutions*

The following risk factors are associated with the nursing diagnosis *Risk for Infection related to the administration of drugs and solutions:* inadequate primary defense, type of operative procedure, inadequate secondary defense, medical conditions and treatments, malnutrition, and extremes of age. (*page 115*)

11. [c] Fluid volume deficit (blood loss) related to the use of heparin

Risk factors associated with the nursing diagnosis *Risk for Fluid Volume Deficit related to the use of heparin* include operative intervention, central nervous system trauma, cardiovascular disease, gender (women older than 60 years of age), gastrointestinal disorders, alterations in vitamin K

absorption, hematological conditions, and other medications or substances. (*page 115*)

12. [a] Mrs. Walter is a 49-year-old woman about to have an emergency surgical procedure because of a motor vehicle accident. There are no family members present, and Mrs. Walter is disoriented and unable to provide a medical history.

Risk factors associated with the nursing diagnosis *Risk for Injury related to hypersensitivity or an adverse reaction to an anticoagulant or antiplatelet agent* include inability of the patient or family member to provide an accurate drug history; history of allergic hypersensitivity to heparin or dextran; heparin resistance resulting from large amounts of fibrin deposits in conditions such as early-stage thrombophlebitis, peritonitis, fever, pleurisy, cancer, myocardial infarction, and extensive operative intervention; and dextran sensitivity. (*page 115*)

13. [c] 84 kg

The nurse should record this weight as 84 kg. The kilogram weight is calculated by dividing 185 by 2.2 (2.2 lb is equal to 1 kg). (*page 114*)

14. [c] *Risk for Decreased Cardiac Output related to toxicity from a local anesthetic*

Risk factors associated with the nursing diagnosis *Risk for Decreased Cardiac Output related to toxicity from a local anesthetic* include history of reaction to the specific agent or a related agent, inability of the patient or family members to provide an accurate drug history, presence of cardiac depressants (which can increase the effect of local anesthetics), and local anesthetics containing epinephrine (which can precipitate arrhythmias). (*page 116*)

15. [a] Osmotic agents can cause hyperglycemia and glycosuria

In diabetes, osmotic agents may cause hyperglycemia and glycosuria. (*page 116*)

16. [b] *Risk for Injury related to allergic reaction to contrast media*

Risk factors associated with the nursing diagnosis of *Risk for Injury related to an allergic reaction to contrast media* include history of allergy to contrast media or a related compound, hypersensitivity to iodine, bronchial asthma, hay fever, and food allergies such as shellfish allergy. (*page 116*)

17. [a] A patient with severe liver disease is a poor candidate for general anesthesia with thiopental sodium (Pentothal) because the final elimination of this drug from the body requires enzymatic breakdown in the liver. (*page 117*)

Preexisting disease states can alter drug metabolism and excretion and cause an unexpected drug response. An example would be a patient with severe liver disease. (*page 117*)

18. [c] Different drugs are taken that act at the same cellular site to produce similar effects

Cross-tolerance can develop with different drugs that act at the same cellular site to produce similar effects. A drug- or alcohol-addicted patient, for example, may prove resistant to a general anesthetic that depresses the central nervous system in much the same way that alcohol does. (*page 117*)

19. [a] Cumulative effect

Cumulative effects can occur when the drugs are ingested at a greater rate than the rate at which they can be eliminated by the patient. If several doses of a drug are taken at regular intervals, accumulation and overdose may result. (*page 117*)

20. [d] Congenital resistance

Congenital resistance is an inborn ability to remain unaffected by certain anti-infective drugs. (*page 118*)

21. [a] Have a direct action on bacteria that will result in destruction or death of the bacteria

A bactericidal agent is a compound that has a direct action on bacteria that results in their destruction or death. (*page 118*)

22. [b] Passive immunity

Passive immunity is a protection against a pathogen and its toxins by transfer of antibodies produced in the body of another individual or animal that has been actively immunized. (*page 118*)

23. [b] The degree of drug effectiveness *may be* affected by psychological factors

Psychological factors influence the patient's willingness to take a medication. The degree of drug effectiveness may be affected by psychological factors. If a patient does not believe that the medication will be effective, chances are that the desired effect will not be achieved. In the case of the placebo effect, a patient who is unaware of the inactive properties of the placebo finds the substance effective for its intended use. (*page 125*)

24. [c] Determine whether the patient has religious beliefs that may influence medication administration and compliance

Religious beliefs and practices play an important role in the patient's perception of health, reaction to illness, and response to medications. By assessing the value-belief pattern, the perioperative nurse obtains data that can influence medication administration and patient compliance. For example, a Seventh-Day Adventist may refuse to ingest narcotics or stimulants because he or she believes that the body is a temple of the Holy Spirit and should be protected from such substances. Jehovah's Witnesses are generally opposed to blood transfusion, although individuals may be persuaded to accept blood in emergencies. Christian Scientists believe that their religion has a healing function, and, although they may seek healthcare for childbirth and fracture, they generally refuse medications, vaccinations, and inoculations. (*page 125*)

25. [d] Harrison Narcotic Act

The Harrison Narcotic Act of 1914 was the first attempt by the federal government to prevent drug abuse in the medical and nursing communities. Later regulations were enacted to control the use of marijuana and to make certain drugs available only by prescription (the Durham-Humphrey Amendment of 1951). Continued abuse of potentially dangerous drugs led to the passage of the Drug Abuse Amendments of 1965. With the continued spread of drug abuse in the 1960s, Congress enacted the Comprehensive Drug Abuse Prevention and Control Act of 1970. (*page 113*)

26. [a] Two

Emergency treatment of infections before the causative agent is known is often begun with a combination of two broad-spectrum drugs. If culture and sensitivity testing indicate that the pathogenic strain is fully susceptible to one of the drugs, the other anti-infective agent may be withdrawn. (*page 118*)

27. [b] Occur when absorbed antibiotics are poorly eliminated and accumulate in the tissue

Although intravenous injection may result in phlebitis, some of the more serious forms of toxicity occur when absorbed antibiotics are poorly eliminated and accumulate in the tissue. (*page 118*)

28. [c] Penicillin

Allergies have been reported with almost every kind of anti-infective drug. Reactions are most common with penicillin. (*page 118*)

29. [b] Prevent implantation and invasion by a specific pathogen

The goal of preoperative and intraoperative chemoprophylaxis is to prevent implantation and invasion by a specific pathogen that is known to be sensitive to the anti-infective agent. (*page 119*)

30. [a] Bacitracin, polymyxin B, and gentamicin

Prostheses, such as penile, testicular, breast, and orthopedic implants, are commonly soaked in an antibiotic solution before being implanted. Commonly used antibiotics include bacitracin, polymyxin B, and gentamicin. (*page 119*)

31. [c] Cefonicid sodium

Cefonicid sodium is often administered before surgery to reduce the incidence of postoperative infections in patients undergoing surgical procedures classified as contaminated or potentially contaminated. It is also given when infections at the operative site present serious risk (e.g., for prosthetic arthroplasty and cardiothoracic and vascular procedures). (*page 119*)

32. [d] Fourth

There are four phases in the process of homeostasis. The first three phases promote blood clotting and prevent blood loss, the fourth phase helps maintain blood fluidity and prevents propagation of clotting beyond the site of injury. This phase is also involved in clot dissolution. (*page 119*)

33. [a] Prevent the extension of clots

Anticoagulants prevent the extension of clots but do not dissolve existing clots. Anticoagulant drugs used for this purpose include heparin and warfarin. (*page 119*)

34. [b] Warfarin

Warfarin acts in the liver to prevent the synthesis of vitamin K–dependent clotting factors and thereby prevents blood coagulation. It does not dissolve existing clots. (*page 119*)

35. [b] Hematocrit

A baseline hematocrit is obtained before initiation of dextran 40 injection and after administration. The nurse should notify the physician if the patient's hematocrit is depressed below 30% by volume. (*page 119*)

36. [c] Thrombus

A thrombus is a solid mass of clotted blood in a vessel or in the heart. (*page 119*)

37. [b] A localized collection of blood in a space, organ, or tissue

A hematoma is a localized collection of blood in a space, organ, or tissue. (*page 119*)

38. [c] To slow down the absorption of the local anesthetic agent

Epinephrine is often added to local anesthetic solutions to slow down the absorption of the drug and to keep the anesthetic at the desired site. This prolongs its blocking effect. (*page 120*)

39. [d] Central nerve block

A central nerve block affects the roots of nerves at various points close to their origin in the spinal cord. (*page 120*)

40. [a] 0.25 mL

One must mix 50 mL of normal saline and 0.25 mL of epinephrine 1:1000 (mL) to get a final epinephrine concentration of 1:200,000. (*page 121*)

41. [a] The patient has glaucoma

Cycloplegic agents are contraindicated in persons with primary glaucoma or a tendency toward glaucoma. (*page 121*)

42. [b] Apply pressure to the inner canthus.

When drops are being instilled, pressure is applied to the inner canthus to lessen systemic absorption of the drug. The solution may otherwise run into the respiratory tract through the lacrimal duct and be absorbed into the bloodstream. (*page 121*)

43. [b] Cholinergic agents

Medications that directly or indirectly cause the sphincter muscles of the iris and of the ciliary body to contract are known as cholinergic agents. (*page 122*)

44. [c] Glaucoma

Parasympathomimetic agents (miotics) are used primarily for topical therapy for glaucoma. (*page 122*)

45. [d] Hydrocortisone

Preparations of polymyxin B, neomycin, and hydrocortisone used for the prevention and treatment of inflammation and superficial bacterial infections of the external auditory canal are contraindicated for patients with herpes simplex, vaccinia, or varicella infection. (*page 124*)

46. [c] Anaphylatoxins and neutrophils release necrotizing enzymes that produce local ischemia and necrosis as a consequence of complement activation

Type III is an autoimmune reaction that is associated with an increased amount of immunoglobulin G. Anaphylatoxins and neutrophils release necrotizing enzymes that produce local ischemia and necrosis as a consequence of complement activation. (*page 127*)

47. [a] Supine

The patient is positioned in a supine or a semi-Fowler position to provide access to the eye and minimize drainage of medication through the lacrimal duct. (*page 131*)

48. [b] Look downward

During installation of eye ointment, the patient should look downward to reduce the blinking reflex. (*page 131*)

49. [b] Allergy to seafood

Protamine sulfate may be contraindicated in patients with a history of seafood allergy because the drug is produced from a purified mixture of simple, low-molecular-weight proteins obtained from the sperm or testes of certain fish species. (*page 133*)

50. [d] Excessive elevation of the container can increase intravascular absorption of the irrigating fluid

The container should not be elevated more than 60 cm above the procedure bed. Excessive elevation can increase intravascular absorption of the irrigating fluid. (*page 135*)

CHAPTER 9

Physiologically Monitoring the Patient

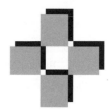

The nurse monitors the patient's physiological status during the operative or invasive procedure. The nurse monitors the patient to prevent ineffective airway clearance and an ineffective breathing pattern, air embolus from intravenous (IV) catheters, local infiltration of IV fluid, fluid volume excess or deficit, hyperthermia or hypothermia, extravasation of IV medication, and cardiodepression related to the administration of local anesthesia. The nurse physiologically monitoring the patient begins by assessing the patient's risk for adverse outcomes related to the monitoring process. Safe monitoring of the patient is essential for the delivery of quality care in the operative and invasive procedure suite. The questions for this chapter will help the reader assess his or her knowledge about

- Managing the patient's airway and breathing pattern
- Managing the patient's fluid intake
- Implementing interventions in response to patient fluid loss
- Maintaining the patient's body temperature
- Monitoring the patient during the administration of IV sedation and local anesthesia

The reference used for this chapter is Phippen, M. L., & Wells, M. P. (1999). *Patient care during operative and invasive procedures.* Philadelphia: W. B. Saunders, pp. 136–146.

✚ Questions

1. Mr. Jones received a peripheral IV of 1000 mL of lactated Ringer's solution at 50 mL/hour. Before the administration of IV sedation, his initial pulse oximeter reading was 94, blood pressure 162/88, heart rate 76, and respirations 22. Following the procedure, Mr. Jones became restless and had a tracheal tug. The nurse should immediately:

   a. Suction Mr. Jones

   b. Turn Mr. Jones on his side

   c. Extend Mr. Jones' head by lifting his jaw

   d. Ventilate Mr. Jones with an Ambu bag

2. When observing for signs of airway obstruction, the nurse may find all of the following except:

   a. Use of accessory muscles during inspiration

   b. Prolonged contraction of abdominal muscles during inspiration

   c. Seesaw movement of the chest and abdomen

   d. Tracheal tug

3. The first step in alleviating an upper airway obstruction is to:

   a. Tilt the head

   b. Inspect the oral cavity

   c. Ventilate the patient with an Ambu bag

   d. Elevate the head of the bed

4. All of the following medications may cause fluid and electrolyte imbalances except:

   a. Furosemide 40 mg orally daily

b. Theophylline 100 mg orally three times a day

c. Prednisone 10 mg orally three times a day

d. Acetazolamide 500 mg orally daily

5. All of the following conditions or disease states may lead to fluid and electrolyte imbalances except:

a. Diabetes

b. Renal failure

c. Chronic obstructive pulmonary disease

d. Burns

6. Ms. Abbott is a 34-year-old librarian woman admitted for an arthroscopy of her left knee. Her blood pressure is 150/88, heart rate 70, and respirations 22. She is 5 feet, 2 inches tall and weighs 282 lb. Which nursing diagnosis is of the highest priority in the immediate postoperative period?

a. *Risk for Infection*

b. *Ineffective Airway Clearance*

c. *Risk for Fluid Volume Overload*

d. *Risk for Oversedation*

7. All of the following conditions may contribute to volume overload except:

a. Cirrhosis of the liver

b. Cushing's syndrome

c. Cardiomyopathy

d. Ulcerative colitis

8. Mr. Smith was trampled by a horse 3 weeks ago and underwent an exploratory laparotomy, bowel resection, and placement of Penrose drains. For the past several days, he has had an increased output from his drains. The surgeon has decided to re-explore Mr. Smith's abdomen. Which nursing diagnosis is of the highest

priority while the patient is in the operating room (OR)?

a. *Risk for Infection*

b. *Ineffective Airway Clearance*

c. *Risk for Fluid Volume Deficit*

d. *Risk for Fluid Volume Overload*

9. The presence of a central IV catheter is a risk factor for which of the following nursing diagnoses?

a. *Risk for Impaired Tissue Integrity related to local infiltration of IV fluid*

b. *Risk for Fluid Volume Excess related to IV therapy*

c. *Risk for Decreased Cardiac Output related to air embolus from IV therapy*

d. *Risk for Fluid Volume Deficit related to IV therapy*

10. Mr. Wheeler is a 74-year-old man scheduled for a total colectomy. During the preoperative nursing assessment, it was noted that Mr. Wheeler is suffering from mild malnutrition. The most appropriate nursing diagnosis is:

a. *Risk for Hypothermia during the operative or invasive procedure*

b. *Risk for Impaired Tissue Integrity related to local infiltration of IV fluid*

c. *Risk for Decreased Cardiac Output related to air embolus*

d. *Risk for Ineffective Breathing Patterns during the operative procedure*

11. The physician has ordered 1500 mL of normal saline to be infused over 24 hours. What is the amount to be infused per hour?

a. 100 mL

b. 62 mL

c. 50 mL

d. 13 mL

12. The physician has ordered 125 mL of lactated Ringer's solution to be infused each hour. The manufacturer states that the tubing will provide 12 drops/mL. How many drops should be infused per minute?

    a. 25 drops

    b. 50 drops

    c. 100 drops

    d. 125 drops

13. The physician order reads: 50 mL of 50% dextrose infused in 2 hours. The manufacturer states that the tubing will provide 60 drops/mL. How many drops should be infused per minute?

    a. 10 drops

    b. 25 drops

    c. 50 drops

    d. 100 drops

14. The physician has ordered 600 mL of normal saline to run at 75 mL/hour. How long will it take for the IV to infuse?

    a. 2 hours

    b. 4 hours

    c. 6 hours

    d. 8 hours

15. An example of an isotonic fluid is:

    a. 0.9% sodium chloride

    b. 0.45% sodium chloride

    c. 5% dextrose in 0.9% sodium chloride

    d. 3% sodium chloride

16. An example of a common hypotonic fluid is:

    a. 5% dextrose in water

    b. 0.45% sodium chloride

    c. 5% dextrose in normal saline

    d. Lactated Ringer's solution

17. What happens when excessive hypertonic fluids are administered?

    a. Circulatory overload

    b. Pulmonary embolism

    c. Mental confusion

    d. Cellular dehydration

18. Mr. Jones complains of shortness of breath and remains restless. His pulse oximeter reading is 90, blood pressure 182/94, heart rate 92, and respirations 32. He has 350 mL remaining in his IV. The nurse should reassess Mr. Jones for:

    a. Possible fluid overload

    b. Possible adverse reaction to IV sedation

    c. Possible lidocaine toxicity

    d. Oxygen toxicity

19. All of the following are signs of hypervolemia except:

    a. Tachycardia

    b. Dyspnea

    c. Hypertension

    d. Flat neck veins

20. The nurse's first intervention for Mr. Jones should be:

    a. Preparing a dose of dilantin

    b. Assisting the anesthesiologist with intubation

    c. Decreasing the oxygen concentration being administered

    d. Slowing the IV flow rate

21. Which of the following amounts of air in an IV line can cause a lethal air embolus?

    a. 10 mL

    b. 20 mL

    c. 30 mL

    d. 50 mL

22. When a large quantity of air is introduced into the circulation, all of the following signs will be present except:

    a. Cyanosis

    b. Anxiety

    c. Hypotension

    d. Decreased cardiac output

23. An air embolus is suspected, the tubing is clamped, the patient is turned to the left side, and placed in Trendelenburg position. These interventions are done to:

    a. Keep the air in the left ventricle

    b. Keep the air in the right ventricle

    c. Keep the air in the left atrium

    d. Keep the air in the right atrium

24. The type and amount of bleeding depend mainly on:

    a. The site of the incision

    b. The type of vessels involved

    c. The length of the surgery

    d. The type of IV fluids administered

25. Hypovolemia is characterized by all of the following except:

    a. Increased peripheral resistance

    b. Increased heart rate

    c. Decreased central venous pressure

    d. Decreased respiratory rate

26. Normal urine output is:

    a. 15 mL/hour

    b. 20 mL/hour

    c. 50 mL/hour

    d. 75 mL/hour

27. A patient is ready for transfer to the post-anesthesia care unit following a colon resection. Prior to leaving the OR suite, the nurse notices that the patient's blood pressure has dropped from 140/72 to 80/54. The first nursing action the nurse should take is to:

    a. Increase the flow of oxygen per mask to 10 L/min

    b. Notify the surgeon

    c. Place the patient in the Trendelenburg position

    d. Recheck the patient's blood pressure and pulse

28. Body temperature is controlled by the:

    a. Thalamus

    b. Hypothalamus

    c. Pituitary gland

    d. Medulla

29. All of the following may affect body temperature except:

    a. Thyroid disease

    b. Diabetes

    c. Hormone imbalance

    d. Sepsis

30. The dissemination of heat through electromagnetic waves coming off the skin is known as:

    a. Conduction

    b. Radiation

    c. Evaporation

    d. Convection

31. The transfer of heat to another object by direct contact as occurs with the use of cooling blankets is known as:

    a. Conduction

    b. Radiation

    c. Evaporation

    d. Convection

32. Why are obese patients at risk for hyperthermia?

    a. They tend to have immature thermal control mechanisms.

    b. They tend to have lower metabolic rates.

    c. Excess fat inhibits release of heat.

    d. Ineffective chemical reaction of metabolism.

33. A decrease in body temperature causes:

    a. Decreased blood pressure, decreased heart rate, vasoconstriction

    b. Increased heart rate, vasodilation, increased blood pressure

    c. Decreased blood pressure, increased heart rate, vasoconstriction

    d. Increased heart rate, vasoconstriction, increased blood pressure

34. Persistent hyperthermia is indicative of a:

    a. Pituitary tumor

    b. Brain stem tumor

    c. Adrenal tumor

    d. Parathyroid tumor

35. Signs of hyperthermia can include all of the following except:

    a. Decreased respirations

    b. Increased heart rate

    c. Seizures

    d. Flushed face

36. Which of the following conditions can predispose a patient to local anesthetic toxicity?

    a. Hyperthyroidism

    b. Cirrhosis of the liver

    c. Chronic obstructive pulmonary disease

    d. Renal failure

37. When administering IV diazepam (Valium), the nurse should:

    a. Dilute the medication with normal saline before administration

    b. Dilute the medication with sterile water before administration

    c. Slowly inject the medication undiluted

    d. Rapidly inject the medication undiluted

38. What age population is most at risk for developing hypothermia during an operative or invasive procedure?

    a. 1–3 months

    b. 11–19 years

    c. 25–49 years

    d. 65–80 years

39. What is the main purpose of IV sedation?

    a. Decrease patient anxiety

    b. Prevent pain

    c. Suppress shivering

    d. Relax muscles

40. Systemic absorption of the local anesthetic can result in:

    a. Increased excitability of the heart

    b. Vasoconstriction

    c. Vasodilatation

    d. Increased contractile force of the heart

✚ Answers

1. [c] Extend Mr. Jones' head by lifting his jaw

Extend the patient's head by lifting the jaw. This increases the distance between the chin and the cervical spine, which puts the muscles that support the chin under tension and pulls the tongue forward. (*page 137*)

2. [b] Prolonged contraction of abdominal muscles during inspiration

Inspiration causes drawing in of parts of the upper chest, the sternum, and the intercostal spaces. Exhalation is characterized by jerky protrusion and prolonged contractions of abdominal muscles. (*page 137*)

3. [b] Inspect the oral cavity

One should open and inspect the mouth for displacement of the tongue and the presence of secretions, blood, and other substances. (*page 137*)

4. [b] Theophylline 100 mg orally three times a day

Assess the use of medications, such as diuretics and adrenocorticosteroid; these may cause fluid and electrolyte imbalances. (*page 138*)

5. [c] Chronic obstructive pulmonary disease

Ingestion of excessive alcohol and nonprescription drugs may interfere with proper nutrition, leading to fluid and electrolyte imbalance. The nurse must not overlook important contributing factors, such as diabetes insipidus, diabetic ketoacidosis, adrenal insufficiency, renal failure, cancer, burns, trauma, pregnancy, and congestive heart failure. (*page 138*)

6. [b] *Ineffective Airway Clearance*

Risk factors associated with ineffective airway and ineffective breathing pattern clearance during the operative or invasive procedure include alteration in level of consciousness caused by IV sedation, history of sleep apnea, pain or fear of pain that may discourage coughing and breathing, obesity, and neuromuscular or musculoskeletal impairment. (*page 139*)

7. [d] Ulcerative colitis

Conditions that contribute to volume overload include excessive fluid or sodium intake, compromised regulatory system, which includes conditions such as congestive heart failure, renal failure, liver disease, stress of the operative or invasive procedure intervention, and Cushing's syndrome; and corticosteroid therapy. (*page 139*)

8. [c] *Risk for Fluid volume deficit*

The nursing diagnosis *Risk for Fluid volume deficit* is associated with the following risk factors: clotting disorder or the use of anticoagulant medications, extremes of age and weight, vomiting, wound drainage, burns, trauma, and hemorrhage. (*page 139*)

9. [c] *Risk for Decreased Cardiac Output related to air embolus from IV therapy*

Risk factors associated with *Risk for Decreased Cardiac Output related to air embolus* from IV therapy include delivery of fluid under pressure and presence of a central IV catheter. (*page 139*)

10. [a] *Risk for Hypothermia during the operative or invasive procedure*

Risk factors associated with the nursing diagnosis *Risk for Hypothermia during the operative and invasive procedure* include trauma or large open wound, exposure of internal organs and body cavities, extremes in age, and malnutrition. (*page 139*)

11. [b] 62 mL

1500 mL (amount of solution to infuse ÷ hours to infuse) = amount to infuse per hour. (*page 140*)

12. [a] 25 drops

125 mL/hour × 12 (drops/mL ÷ 60 minutes/hour) = 25 drops/minute. (*page 140*)

13. [b] 25 drops

25 mL/hour × 60 (drops/mL ÷ 60 minutes/hour) = 25 drops/minute. (*page 140*)

14. [d] 8 hours

600 (amount of solution) ÷ 75 (amount to infuse per hour) = 8 hours. (*page 140*)

15. [a] 0.9% sodium chloride

Commonly used isotonic fluids include 5% dextrose in water, normal saline (0.9% sodium chloride), and lactated Ringer's solution. Isotonic fluids increase the extracellular fluid volume, which can cause circulatory overload. (*page 140*)

16. [b] 0.45% sodium chloride

Commonly used hypotonic fluids include half-normal saline (0.45% sodium chloride) and 2.5% dextrose in water. (*page 140*)

17. [d] Cellular dehydration

If excessive hypertonic fluids are administered, cellular dehydration can result. (*page 140*)

18. [a] Possible fluid overload

If not corrected, hypervolemia can lead to congestive heart failure, which is manifested by dyspnea, neck vein distention, tachycardia, hypertension or hypotension, and cardiac ischemia. (*page 141*)

19. [d] Flat neck veins

Hypervolemia is manifested by dyspnea, neck vein distention, tachycardia, hypotension or hypertension, and cardiac ischemia. Laboratory findings may include a low hematocrit and low total protein count. (*page 141*)

20. [d] Slowing the IV flow rate

If symptoms of fluid excess develop, the rate of the infusion should be slowed at once and the physician notified. The nurse should monitor vital signs and electrolyte values and report the findings to the physician and document them on the operative or invasive procedure record. (*page 141*)

21. [d] 50 mL

Although small amounts of air are not hazardous, a volume of 50 mL can be lethal when delivered as a bolus. (*page 141*)

22. [b] Anxiety

The result of a large quantity of air introduced into the circulation is a significant decrease in cardiac output, which can lead to hypotension and cardiac arrest. (*page 141*)

23. [d] Keep the air in the right atrium

If an air embolus is suspected, the tubing should be clamped and the patient should be placed on his or her left side in the Trendelenburg position. These interventions keep the air in the right atrium, where it can be absorbed or removed through a central venous catheter. (*page 142*)

24. [b] The type of vessels involved

The type and amount of bleeding depend on the type of vessels involved. Capillary hemorrhage is characterized by a slow, general ooze. Venous hemorrhage bubbles out quickly and is dark. Arterial hemorrhage is bright red and spurts out with each heartbeat. (*page 142*)

25. [d] Decreased respiratory rate

Hypovolemia is characterized by a fall in venous pressure, a rise in peripheral resistance, and tachycardia. (*page 142*)

26. [d] 50 mL/hour

Normal urine output is 50 mL/hour. An output of 0.5 mL/kg/hour is suggestive of inadequate volume replacement or cardiac failure. (*page 142*)

27. [c] Place the patient in the Trendelenburg position

If hypotension occurs, the patient is placed in the supine or Trendelenburg position and oxygen, fluids, and medications are administered as needed. (*page 142*)

28. [b] Hypothalamus

Body temperature is controlled by the hypothalamus, which acts as the body's thermostat. The hypothalamus mediates temperature control through secretion of thyroid-stimulating hormone–releasing hormone, which initiates a series of actions that result in heat production and conservation. (*page 143*)

29. [b] Diabetes

Increases in metabolic rate, as occur with malignant hyperthermia, thyroid disease, or imbalances of hormonal production, may alter temperature. (*page 143*)

30. [b] Radiation

Radiation is the dissemination of heat through electromagnetic waves coming off the skin. (*page 143*)

31. [a] Conduction

Conduction is the transfer of heat to another object by direct contact, as occurs with the use of a cooling blanket. (*page 143*)

32. [c] Excess fat inhibits release of heat.

Individuals who are overweight may be at risk for hyperthermia because of excess fat, which inhibits release of heat. (*page 143*)

33. [b] Increased heart rate, vasodilation, increased blood pressure

A patient with hypothermia may exhibit arrhythmias, ventricular irritability, increased bleeding tendency, changes in arterial blood gas values, alterations in acid-base balance, and an increase in heart rate, stroke volume, arterial blood pressure, cardiac output, and oxygen consumption. (*page 143*)

34. [b] Brain stem tumor

Persistent hyperthermia may indicate brain stem damage. Additionally, the presence of intraventricular blood can also cause temperature elevations. (*page 144*)

35. [a] Decreased respirations

The patient with hyperthermia may complain of headache, thirst, general malaise, and palpitations. Overt signs can include increased body temperature, flushed skin, warm skin, increased respirations, tachycardia, seizures, and convulsions. (*page 144*)

36. [b] Cirrhosis of the liver

Patients with hepatic disease may have ineffective metabolism, which may result in toxic responses, even with normal doses. (*page 145*)

37. [c] Slowly inject the medication undiluted

When administering IV drugs, one must avoid mixing or diluting the drug with other drugs or solutions in the same syringe or container. The nurse injects the drug slowly, taking time to assess the patient's response to the medication. The dose can then be individualized and titrated. (*page 145*)

38. [a] 1–3 months

Children less than 3 months of age are at particular risk because hypothermia can induce reopening of fetal circulation, with reluctant acidosis and hypoxemia, which becomes a circular pattern of events that is difficult to reverse. (*page 143*)

39. [a] Decrease patient anxiety

The primary purpose of IV sedation is to decrease the patient's fears and anxiety related to the procedure. (*page 144*)

40. [c] Vasodilatation

Systemic absorption of the local anesthetic can result in vasodilatation and cardiac depression. (*page 146*)

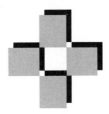

CHAPTER 10

Monitoring and Controlling the Environment

Monitoring and controlling the environment refers to those activities performed by the nurse that promote the safety and well-being of the patient during an operative or invasive procedure. The nurse protects the patient from hazards within the environment and provides an environment that promotes infection control. The questions for this chapter will help the reader assess his or her knowledge about

- Identifying the patient's risk for adverse outcomes related to monitoring and controlling the environment
- Regulating temperature and humidity
- Ensuring electrical safety
- Ensuring fire safety
- Ensuring environmental air quality
- Monitoring the sensory environment
- Ensuring radiation safety
- Ensuring laser safety
- Maintaining suite traffic patterns
- Preventing latex exposure to sensitive patients and staff
- Performing environmental sanitation
- Sterilizing instruments, supplies, and equipment

The reference used for this chapter is Phippen, M. L., & Wells, M. P. (1999). *Patient care during operative and invasive procedures.* Philadelphia: W. B. Saunders, pp. 147–166.

✚ Questions

1. The perioperative nurse is responsible for monitoring room temperature and humidity levels. A relative humidity of _____ inhibits bacterial growth and decreases the potential for static electricity.

    a. 40%–60%

    b. 50%–65%

    c. 50%–60%

    d. 45%–55%

2. A room temperature of _____ inhibits bacterial growth.

    a. 68°–76°F (20°–24.4°C)

    b. 65°–76°F (18.3°–24.4°C)

    c. 68°–78°F (20°–25.5°C)

    d. 65°–78°F (18.3°–25.5°C)

3. Before the first case of the day is started, a baseline reading of the operating room (OR) temperature and humidity level should be taken. Except in extenuating circumstances such as an emergency or when the room temperature is raised to accommodate a patient at risk for alteration in body temperature, when the temperature or humidity is not within normal range (as described in questions 1 and 2), who should be notified?

    a. Infection control nurse

    b. Hospital engineer

    c. Infection control nurse, OR manager, and hospital engineer

    d. OR manager

4. What factors should the perioperative nurse consider when assessing the patient for temperature monitoring and control devices?

    a. The patient's physical status, type of anesthesia planned, ambient room temperature, length and type of surgical procedure

b. The patient's age, the patient's physical and emotional status, type of anesthesia planned, static room temperature, length of surgical procedure

c. The patient's age, the patient's physical status, type of anesthesia planned, ambient room temperature, length and type of surgical procedure

d. The patient's age, type of anesthesia planned, and ambient room temperature

5. Patients at risk for experiencing intraoperative alterations in body temperature should have their temperature monitored with an appropriate thermometer. Before using the thermometer, the perioperative nurse should:

a. Test it according to the manufacturer's instructions to ensure that it is in working order

b. Test it according to hospital policy and procedure

c. Insert the thermometer before the patient is anesthetized

d. Wipe the thermometer with a germicidal solution to prevent cross-contamination

6. The perioperative nurse should insert a rectal thermometer how far into the rectum?

a. ½–1 inches

b. ½–1½ inches

c. 1–2 inches

d. 1–2¾ inches

7. The perioperative nurse conserves the patient's body heat by:

(1) Covering the patient with warm blankets

(2) Warming preparation solutions, intravenous infusions, blood, and irrigating solutions

(3) Moistening sponges with warm saline before handing them to the surgeon

(4) Blotting the patient's skin dry after the skin preparation

a. (1) and (2)

b. (1) and (4)

c. (2), (3), and (4)

d. All of the above

8. The perioperative nurse provides alternative methods of temperature regulation:

a. If the patient is identified as being at high risk for altered body temperature

b. According to policy and procedure

c. If the surgeon orders the application of temperature regulation devices

d. If the anesthesiologist orders the application of temperature regulation devices

9. What nursing diagnosis is most appropriate for a neonate having surgery during the first 24 hours of life?

a. *Risk for Injury related to supine positioning*

b. *Risk for Hyperthermia*

c. *Risk for Postoperative Urinary Tract Infection*

d. *Risk for Altered Body Temperature during the intraoperative period*

10. Perioperative nursing interventions for the neonate include the use of warming blankets and heat lamps. While excellent sources of heat, these devices also place the neonate at risk for:

a. Hyperthermia

b. Thermal injury

c. Electrical injury

d. Impaired tissue integrity

11. The perioperative nurse conserves the neonate's body heat by:

    (1) Covering the head with a surgical cap

    (2) Encasing the extremities in stockinet

    (3) Wrapping the extremities with Webril

    (4) Wrapping the extremities with aluminum foil

    a. (3) and (4)

    b. (2) and (3)

    c. (1) and (4)

    d. (1) and (2)

12. What does the perioperative nurse document concerning the use of thermoregulation devices?

    a. Types of thermoregulation devices used and skin conditions before and after the procedure

    b. Types of thermoregulation devices used, the skin conditions before and after the procedure, and the patient's baseline temperature

    c. Patient's baseline temperature

    d. Types of thermoregulation devices used and the patient's baseline temperature

13. What is the purpose of an isolated power system?

    a. Monitors for current leaks and grounding during power surges

    b. Decreases the risk of accidental grounding of persons in contact with a hot wire

    c. Prevents shock, cardiac fibrillation, or burns from electrical current flowing through the patient's body to ground

    d. Prevents accidental grounding of persons in contact with a hot wire

14. If the isolated power system is functional, the alarm sounds only when faulty equipment is plugged into ungrounded circuits. If this occurs, the perioperative nurse should:

    a. Notify the supervisor

    b. Immediately disconnect the electrosurgical generator

    c. Shut off and unplug the last electrical device plugged into the electrical system

    d. Notify the biomedical engineering department

15. If, after action is taken, the alarm light of the isolated monitor remains lit, the perioperative nurse should:

    a. Unplug the electrical equipment until the defective device is identified

    b. Send the device to the bioengineering department for repair

    c. Replace the electrosurgical generator

    d. Check the electrosurgical dispersive pad to ensure that it is still firmly attached to the patient

16. Before using electrical equipment, the perioperative nurse should:

    (1) Ensure that routine inspections occur at least every 6 months along with the scheduled preventive maintenance

    (2) Inspect the equipment for frayed cords, loose wires, and lack of secure connections

    (3) Test the electrical units before use for functioning audio alarms and lights

    (4) Check outlets and switch plates for damage

    a. (1), (2), and (3)

    b. (1), (3), and (4)

    c. (2) and (3)

    d. (2), (3), and (4)

17. Mrs. Smith is a 65-year-old woman scheduled for a hemicolectomy. She has a

known diagnosis of lupus erythematosus. The most appropriate nursing diagnosis would be:

a. *Risk for Injury related to the use of laser instruments*

b. *Risk for Injury related to radiation exposure*

c. *Risk for Infection*

d. *Risk for Altered Body Temperature*

18. Mrs. Hall is scheduled to have a revision of her ileostomy. She has many food allergies, such as avocados, kiwi, bananas, melon, figs, tomatoes, and celery. The most appropriate nursing diagnosis for Mrs. Hall would be:

a. *Risk for Injury secondary to latex exposure*

b. *Risk for Infection*

c. *Risk for Injury related to allergies to anesthesia agents*

d. *Risk for Impaired Skin Integrity related to malnutrition*

19. Which of the following statements are true concerning electrical safety practices?

(1) Exercise care when placing receptacles containing liquid on top of electrical equipment.

(2) During cleaning procedures, avoid saturating electrical equipment with liquid.

(3) Spray liquid only on horizontal surfaces of equipment and wipe air vents with a clean, damp cloth.

(4) During the procedure, ensure that foot pedals that activate electrical equipment remain dry.

(5) Carefully roll heavy equipment (beds, x-ray machines) over electrical cords to prevent damage.

(6) Avoid using extension cords. If extension cords are necessary, use only those that are designed for

heavy-duty use and approved by the hospital biomedical engineering department.

a. (1), (4), and (6)

b. (2), (4), and (6)

c. (3), (5), and (6)

d. (2), (3), and (5)

20. When managing a small fire in the operative and invasive procedure room, the first step would be to:

a. Evacuate the room

b. Use a fire extinguisher

c. Smother the burning material with a dripping-wet sponge

d. Stop the flow of breathing gases to the patient

21. There is an airway fire during a tracheostomy. The first thing to be done would be to:

a. Remove the endotracheal tube

b. Smother the fire with a dripping wet sponge

c. Disconnect breathing circuit from the endotracheal tube

d. Evacuate the room

22. A patient having an endoscopic procedure with the use of electrosurgery is at what additional risk?

a. Absorption of carbon monoxide formed in the cavity

b. Bronchiolitis from the smoke

c. Exposure to hydrogen cyanide

d. Exposure to visible and odious smoke

23. Fear, a common reaction in many surgical patients, is often related to:

a. Knowledge deficit

b. Anticipatory anxiety

c. Self-esteem disturbance

d. Potential body image disturbance

24. The perioperative nurse begins preoperative teaching by assessing the patient's:

a. Level of anxiety

b. Risk for body image disturbance

c. Level of self-esteem

d. Knowledge level about the surgical environment

25. Sensory stimuli in the surgical environment often contribute to a patient's feelings of fear and anxiety. An appropriate intervention to decrease sensory stimuli is:

a. Administration of an amnesic drug

b. Patient teaching

c. Reassurance

d. Speaking loudly so as not to hide information from the patient

26. Nursing personnel should wear radiation badges:

a. Clipped to the chest

b. Clipped on the apron belt

c. On the scrub shirt sleeve

d. At the neckline

27. During surgery, Mr. Jones will have abdominal radiographs taken. Anticipating this, the perioperative nurse places a lead collar over Mr. Jones':

a. Chest

b. Neck

c. Testicles

d. Chest and neck

28. How often should the OR manager have leaded protective devices radiographically inspected for cracks and structural integrity?

a. Monthly

b. Annually

c. Biannually

d. Bimonthly

29. After using them, the perioperative nurse stores protective devices by:

a. Folding and placing them on the portable x-ray unit

b. Laying them flat or hanging them on an appropriate rack

c. Returning them to the radiology department

d. Placing them in the appropriate storage cabinet

30. After implantation of radioactive materials into a patient, the perioperative nurse instructs:

a. Recovery or floor personnel that they will receive a patient with radioactive implants

b. The radiology department that the procedure is completed

c. The family to wear protective devices while visiting the patient

d. An orderly to take the container used to transport material to the OR back to the nuclear medicine department

31. When operating a laser, the perioperative nurse should:

a. Follow hospital policy and procedure

b. Follow the manufacturer's recommendations and instructions

c. Check and test the laser equipment after use

d. Cover the eyes of the anesthetized patient with appropriate protective glasses

32. Which of the following is *not* a laser safety device?

a. Protective wear specific for laser beam

b. Wet gauze or cloth towels

c. Special anesthesia endotracheal equipment for head and neck surgery

d. Reflective instruments

33. Which response is *incorrect* concerning the use of a laser during surgery?

a. Use laser-retardant drapes around the operative site.

b. Keep towels and sponges surrounding the target tissue wet at all times.

c. Have a carbon dioxide fire extinguisher readily available during a laser procedure.

d. Have a bucket of water in the room in case flammable materials are ignited.

34. Laser documentation includes all of the following *except* the:

a. Name of the hospital laser safety officer

b. Type of laser used

c. Lens used

d. Wattage used for the procedure

35. In the restricted zone, personnel must wear appropriate scrub attire and surgical masks. This zone includes all of the following areas *except:*

a. Substerile areas

b. The instrument-processing area

c. Sterile core areas

d. Operating rooms

36. Methods to decrease potential airborne contamination include all of the following *except:*

a. Keeping traffic flow into and out of the room to a minimum

b. Keeping doors closed

c. Barring personnel with skin infections from restricted areas unless they wear gown and gloves

d. Barring sick personnel from working in restricted areas

37. Methods to decrease potential contamination from outside environmental sources include all of the following *except:*

a. Damp dusting or wiping down with a germicidal solution all equipment brought into the surgical suite

b. Transporting clean and sterile items to the OR in an enclosed container or on a covered cart

c. Cleaning patient transport gurneys after each use

d. Removing protective coverings after supply carts are brought into the OR

38. The most common clinical reaction associated with latex is:

a. Contact dermatitis

b. Irritant contact dermatitis

c. Allergic contact dermatitis

d. Immediate allergic reaction

39. The perioperative nurse should implement the same environmental sanitation protocols for every surgical procedure *except:*

a. Open bowel procedures with spillage

b. Procedures contaminated with pus

c. Procedures on patients with confirmed human immunodeficiency virus infection

d. None of the above

40. Before the first scheduled surgery, the perioperative nurse should:

a. Damp dust all horizontal and vertical surfaces, including furniture, surgical lights, and equipment, with a clean, lint-free cloth moistened in a hospital-grade disinfectant

b. Damp dust all horizontal surfaces, including furniture, and equipment, with a clean, lint-free moist cloth

c. Damp dust all horizontal surfaces, including furniture, surgical lights, and equipment, with a clean, lint-free cloth moistened in a hospital-grade disinfectant

d. Dust all horizontal surfaces, including furniture, surgical lights, and equipment, with a clean cloth

41. When organic debris falls from the sterile field, the perioperative nurse should perform the following tasks *except:*

a. Remove the debris with a disposable cloth

b. Saturate the area with a germicidal solution

c. Remove the debris with a disposable cloth and cover the area with a clean cloth

d. Discard the contaminated cloths into an impervious container

42. Which statement is true?

a. Deposit soiled sponges in a plastic-lined bucket.

b. Ensure that soiled sponges placed on a draped table or spread on an impervious barrier on the floor are at least 5 feet from the sterile field.

c. If a contaminated instrument is required for immediate use, before sterilization, rinse all blood off the instrument with cold water.

d. If a reusable suction container is used, rinse after each use with cold water.

43. Which statement is false?

a. At the end of the procedure, clean all horizontal surfaces, and surfaces that have come in immediate contact with a patient or patient secretions, with germicidal solution.

b. If hospital policy dictates disposal of suction container fluids, empty contents of the suction container into a flushing hopper.

c. Use protective eyewear, masks or face shield, apron or gown, and gloves when disposing of suction container fluids.

d. Recap needles or disassemble disposable syringes when disposing of sharps.

44. Which statement is false?

a. Remove gown and gloves before leaving the OR.

b. After removing trash, linen, and instruments, flood the floors with a germicidal detergent and wet vacuum.

c. When cleaning the OR bed, wipe all surfaces and mattress pads with a lint-free cloth soaked in germicidal detergent.

d. After cleaning overhead surgical spotlights, wipe the surgical light reflector shields with distilled water to remove detergent film.

45. Which statement is true?

a. Only instruments placed on the Mayo tray during the procedure should be decontaminated.

b. Instruments opened during the procedure should be decontaminated.

c. Instruments placed on the back table during the procedure and *unused* do not need to be decontaminated.

d. Instruments opened and used during the procedure should be decontaminated.

46. During the surgical procedure, the scrub person removes gross blood and other debris from instruments by wiping:

a. Or prerinsing the instruments with normal saline

b. The instruments with a moist radiopaque 4 × 8 sponge

c. Or prerinsing the instruments with sterile water

d. The instruments with a moist laparotomy sponge

47. After the procedure is completed, the scrub person:

a. Opens and places used instruments in normal saline

b. Transports used supplies and equipment to the decontamination section of the instrument-processing area in a way that avoids contamination of personnel or any area of the hospital

c. Opens and places all instruments in distilled water

d. Transports all supplies and equipment to the decontamination section of the instrument-processing area in a way that avoids contamination of personnel or any area of the hospital

48. After the procedure, if a washer-sterilizer is not available, instruments should be:

a. Placed in the sonic cleaner before handling

b. Flash sterilized before handling

c. Rinsed in distilled water and soaked in glutaraldehyde before handling

d. Submerged and washed manually in an appropriate germicidal solution

49. Which of the following statements is true?

a. After the initial washing of general instruments, the instruments are placed in an ultrasonic cleaner, which removes debris that may have been missed.

b. Before the initial washing of general instruments, the instruments are placed in an ultrasonic cleaner, which removes debris that may have been missed by the scrub person.

c. Before manual washing of general instruments, the instruments are placed in an ultrasonic cleaner, which removes debris that may have been missed by the scrub person.

d. After the initial washing of general instruments, the instruments are assembled and wrapped for processing.

50. Dissimilar metals, such as copper, stainless steel, and brass, should not be combined in the:

a. Ultrasonic cleaner

b. Flash autoclave

c. Gravity displaced autoclave

d. Ethylene oxide sterilizer

51. Instruments that have been in the ultrasonic cleaner should:

a. Not be lubricated with a water-soluble solution

b. Be sterilized as soon as possible

c. Be lubricated with a water-soluble solution and then allowed to dry

d. Be lubricated with a water-soluble solution and then rinsed with sterile water

52. Which of the following statements concerning preparation of instruments for sterilization are true?

(1) Box locks of instruments are opened for the sterilization cycle.

(2) Heavy instruments should be placed in the bottom of the sterilizing tray.

(3) Delicate instruments are wrapped separately and placed on the top of the heavy instruments.

(4) The weight of instrument sets should not exceed approximately 20 lb.

(5) When being sterilized with ethylene oxide, items with lumina, such as tubes, needles,

and drains, should be flushed with distilled water before being placed in the tray.

a. (1), (2), and (3)

b. (1), (2), and (4)

c. (3), (4), and (5)

d. All of the above

53. Which statement is true concerning the loading of items for steam sterilization?

a. Basins and solid-bottomed trays are placed flat during the sterilization cycle.

b. Flat packages are placed on the sterilizer shelf horizontally.

c. Linen packages and packages containing metal should be sterilized separately.

d. Linen packages go on the top level of the sterilizer and metal on the bottom when running a mixed load.

54. After the sterilizer cart is removed from the autoclave:

a. It should be placed near air vents or fans to accelerate cooling

b. It should not be placed near air vents or fans to avoid the possibility of condensation

c. It should not be placed near air vents or fans to avoid the possibility of contamination

d. The items from the sterilizing cart are removed and placed on an empty cart for cooling

55. Which of the following statements is true concerning flash sterilization?

a. When flashing 11 or more metal instruments, the instruments are sterilized for 10 minutes at or above 270°F.

b. When flashing metal instruments, the instruments are sterilized for 3 minutes at or above 270°F.

c. Sterilize porous items or mixed porous-nonporous items for 10 minutes at or above 270°F and dry for 20 minutes.

d. Specialty items are never flash sterilized.

56. Before ethylene oxide sterilization, items must be thoroughly clean and dry. Otherwise, the combination of water and ethylene oxide forms a toxic substance, which is:

a. Ethylene glycan

b. Ethyl glycol

c. Ethylene glycol

d. Ethylene gluconate

57. After the ethylene oxide sterilization cycle is complete, the sterilizer door is opened as soon as possible after completion of the sterilization cycle to:

a. Decrease ethylene oxide vapor build-up

b. Prevent vacuum lock

c. Decrease ethylene glycol vapor build-up

d. Accelerate aeration time

58. One should avoid touching ethylene oxide sterilized items when transferring the items to the aerator because:

a. The items have not been aerated

b. Ethylene oxide can burn the skin

c. Wrappers retain ethylene glycol

d. Ethylene oxide vapors build up

59. The Bowie-Dick test is carried out to determine the:

a. Efficacy of the vacuum system of a prevacuum sterilizer

b. Efficiency of sterilization of a prevacuum sterilizer

c. Efficacy of the air removal system of a gravity displacement sterilizer

d. Efficacy and efficiency of the vacuum system and sterilization cycle of a prevacuum sterilizer

60. Which of the following statements is true concerning biological sterilization indicators?

(1) *Bacillus stearothermophilus* is used to test ethylene oxide sterilizers.

(2) *Bacillus subtilis* is used to test steam sterilizers.

(3) *Bacillus subtilis* is used to test ethylene oxide sterilizers.

(4) *Bacillus stearothermophilus* is used to test steam sterilizers.

a. (1) and (3)

b. (2) and (3)

c. (1) and (4)

d. (3) and (4)

✛ Answers

1. [c] 50%–60%

The perioperative nurse is responsible for monitoring room temperature and humidity levels. A relative humidity of 50%–60% inhibits bacterial growth and decreases the potential for static electricity. (*page 147*)

2. [a] 68°–76°F

A room temperature of 68°–76°F (20°–24.4°C) inhibits bacterial growth and decreases the potential for static electricity. (*page 147*)

3. [d] OR manager

Before the first case of the day is started, a baseline reading of the OR temperature and humidity level should be taken. Except in extenuating circumstances such as a emergency or when the room temperature is raised to accommodate a patient at risk for alteration in body temperature, when the temperature or humidity is not within normal range (as described in questions 1 and 2), the OR manager should be notified. (*page 147*)

4. [d] The patient's age, type of anesthesia planned, and ambient room temperature

The perioperative nurse should consider the following factors when assessing the patient for temperature monitoring or control devices: the patient's age, the patient's physical status, type of anesthesia planned, ambient room temperature, and length and type of surgical procedure. (*page 147*)

5. [a] Test it according to manufacturer's instructions to ensure that it is in working order

Patients at risk for experiencing intraoperative alterations in body temperature should have their temperature monitored with an appropriate thermometer. Before using the thermometer, the perioperative nurse should test it according to the manufacturer's instructions to ensure that it is in working order. (*page 148*)

6. [c] 1–2 inches

When inserting a rectal thermometer, the perioperative nurse inserts the thermometer 1–2 inches into the rectum. (*page 148*)

7. [d] All of the above

The perioperative nurse conserves the patient's body heat by covering the patient with warm blankets; warming preparation solutions, intravenous infusions, blood, and irrigating solutions, moistening sponges with warm saline before handing them to the surgeon; and blotting the patient's skin dry after the skin preparation. (*page 148*)

8. [a] If the patient is identified as being at high risk for altered body temperature

The perioperative nurse provides alternative methods of temperature regulation if the patient is identified as being at high risk for altered body temperature. These methods include warming and cooling blankets and external heat sources. (*page 148*)

9. [d] *Risk for Altered Body Temperature during the intraoperative period*

A neonate having surgery during the first 24 hours of life is at high risk for altered body temperature during the intraoperative period. The neonate's body heat is conserved by covering the head with a stockinet cap and encasing the extremities with Webril. (*page 148*)

10. [b] Thermal injury

Perioperative nursing interventions for a neonate at risk for altered body temperature during the intraoperative period include the use of warming blankets and heat lamps as good sources of external heat. (*page 148*)

11. [b] (2) and (3)

The perioperative nurse conserves the neonate's body heat by encasing the extremities in stockinet and wrapping the extremities with Webril. (*page 148*)

12. [b] Types of thermoregulation devices used, the skin conditions before and after the procedure, and the patient's baseline temperature

The perioperative nurse documents the types of thermoregulation devices used, the skin conditions before and after the procedure, and the patient's baseline temperature. (*page 148*)

13. [d] Prevents accidental grounding of persons in contact with a hot wire

The isolated power system prevents accidental grounding of persons in contact with a hot wire. The isolated power system continually monitors for current leaks and grounding and thus reduces the hazard of shock, cardiac fibrillation, or burns. (*page 148*)

14. [c] Shut off and unplug the last electrical device plugged into the electrical system

If the isolated power system is functional, the alarm sounds only when faulty equipment is plugged into ungrounded circuits. If this occurs, the perioperative nurse should shut off and unplug the last electrical device plugged into the electrical system. (*page 148*)

15. [a] Unplug the electrical equipment until the defective device is identified

In the event that the alarm of the isolated monitor sounds and the alarm light remains lit after action has been taken, the perioperative should continue to unplug electrical equipment until the defective device is identified. (*page 148*)

16. [d] Inspect equipment for frayed cords, test the electrical units before use, and check outlets and switch plates for damage

Before using electrical equipment, the perioperative nurse should inspect the equipment for frayed cords, loose wires, and lack of secure connections; test the electrical units before use for functioning audio alarms and lights; and check outlets and switch plates for damage. (*page 150*)

17. [c] *Risk for Infection*

Risk factors associated with the nursing diagnosis *Risk for Infection* include impaired skin integrity, chronic disease leading to suppressed immunity (lupus erythematosus), impaired tissue perfusion, high white blood cell count, low platelet count, and anemia. (*page 149*)

18. [a] *Risk for Injury secondary to latex exposure*

Risk factors associated with the nursing diagnosis *Risk for Injury secondary to latex exposure* include spina bifida and congenital genitourinary abnormalities; occupations in the rubber industry; multiple previous procedures; food allergies to bananas, avocados, chestnuts, apricots, kiwi, papayas, passion fruit, pineapple, melon, figs, grapes, potatoes, tomatoes, and celery. (*page 150*)

19. [b] (2), (4), and (6)

When using electrical equipment, the perioperative nurse avoids saturating electrical equipment with liquid during cleaning procedures, ensures that foot pedals that activate electrical equipment remain dry, and avoids using extension cords. (*page 151*)

20. [c] Smother the burning material with a dripping-wet sponge

When managing small fires, one should smother burning material with a dripping-wet sponge or towel. For fire on or near draping material, the drapes are immediately removed. Smoldering embers may be hidden beneath drapes and can result in another flareup. (*page 154*)

21. [c] Disconnect breathing circuit from the endotracheal tube

The steps to follow in the event of an airway fire are to disconnect the breathing circuit from the endotracheal tube, remove the endotracheal tube, obtain assistance to extinguish the fire, ensure that all the tube pieces are removed, care for the patient, re-establish the airway, and examine and treat the patient. (*page 154*)

22. [a] Absorption of the carbon monoxide formed in the cavity

An additional risk for patients having endoscopic procedures with the use of electrosurgery or laser is absorption of the carbon monoxide formed in the cavity. (*page 155*)

23. [a] Knowledge deficit

Fear, a common reaction in many surgical patients, is often related to knowledge deficit. (*page 155*)

24. [d] Knowledge level about the surgical environment

The perioperative nurse begins preoperative teaching by assessing the patient's knowledge level about the surgical environment. (*page 155*)

25. [b] Patient teaching

Sensory stimuli in the surgical environment often contribute to a patient's feelings of fear and anxiety. An appropriate intervention to decrease sensory stimuli is patient teaching. (*page 155*)

26. [d] At the neckline

Nursing personnel should wear radiation badges at the neckline. (*page 156*)

27. [c] Testicles

If abdominal radiographs are to be taken during surgery, the perioperative nurse places a lead collar over the patient's testicles. (*page 156*)

28. [c] Biannually

The OR manager has leaded protective devices radiographically inspected biannually for cracks and structural integrity. (*page 156*)

29. [b] Laying them flat or hanging them on an appropriate rack

After use, the perioperative nurse stores protective devices by laying them flat or hanging them on an appropriate rack. (*page 156*)

30. [a] Recovery or floor personnel that they will receive a patient with radioactive implants

After implantation of radioactive materials into a patient, the perioperative nurse notifies recovery or floor personnel that they will receive a patient with radioactive implants. (*page 156*)

31. [b] Follow manufacturer's recommendations and instructions

When operating a laser, the perioperative nurse should follow the manufacturer's recommendations and instructions. (*page 156*)

32. [d] Reflective instruments

Reflective instruments are not used in laser surgery. Instruments should be nonreflective. (*page 157*)

33. [c] Have a carbon dioxide fire extinguisher readily available during a laser procedure.

The perioperative nurse should have a fire extinguisher readily available during a laser procedure. (*page 157*)

34. [a] Name of the hospital laser safety officer

The hospital laser safety officer would not be documented unless he or she were part of the operative or nursing care teams. (*page 157*)

35. [b] The instrument-processing area

The instrument-processing area is part of the semirestricted zone. (*page 157*)

36. [c] Barring personnel with skin infections from restricted areas unless they wear gown and gloves

Personnel with skin infections should *not* work in a restricted area. (*page 157*)

37. [d] Removing protective coverings after supply carts are brought into the OR

Protective coverings should be removed before supply carts are brought into the OR. (*page 157*)

38. [a] Contact dermatitis

The most common clinical reaction associated with latex and its additives is contact dermatitis. (*page 158*)

39. [d] None of the above

Every procedure should be considered contaminated. Therefore, the perioperative nurse should implement the same environmental sanitation protocols for every surgical procedure. (*page 159*)

40. [c] Damp dust all horizontal surfaces, including furniture, surgical lights, and equipment, with a clean, lint-free cloth moistened in a hospital-grade disinfectant.

Before the first scheduled surgery, the perioperative nurse should damp dust all horizontal surfaces, including furniture, surgical lights, and equipment, with a clean, lint-free cloth moistened in a hospital-grade disinfectant. (*page 159*)

41. [c] Remove the debris with a disposable cloth and cover the area with a clean cloth

When organic debris falls from the sterile field, the perioperative nurse removes the debris with a disposable cloth, saturates the area with a germicidal solution, cleans the area with a clean cloth, and discards the con-

taminated cloths into an impervious container. (*page 160*)

42. [a] Deposit soiled sponges in a plastic-lined bucket

The perioperative nurse should deposit soiled sponges in a plastic-lined bucket. (*page 160*)

43. [d] Recap needles or disassemble disposable syringes when disposing of sharps.

The perioperative nurse or surgical technologist does not recap needles or disassemble disposable syringes when disposing of sharps. (*page 160*)

44. [d] After cleaning overhead surgical spotlights, wipe the surgical light reflector shields with distilled water to remove detergent film.

After overhead surgical spotlights have been cleaned, the light reflector shield should be wiped with 70% isopropyl alcohol to remove detergent film. (*page 160*)

45. [b] Instruments opened during the procedure should be decontaminated.

All instrument trays and instruments opened during the procedure should be decontaminated. (*page 161*)

46. [c] Or prerinsing the instruments with sterile water

During the surgical procedure, the scrub person removes gross blood and other debris from instruments by wiping or prerinsing the instruments with sterile water. (*page 161*)

47. [b] Transports used supplies and equipment to the decontamination section of the instrument-processing area in a way that avoids contamination of personnel or any area of the hospital

After the procedure is completed, the scrub person transports used supplies and equipment to the decontamination section of the instrument-processing area in a way that avoids contamination of personnel or any area of the hospital. (*page 161*)

48. [d] Submerged and washed manually in an appropriate germicidal solution

After the procedure, if a washer-sterilizer is not available, instruments should be submerged and washed manually in an appropriate germicidal solution. (*page 161*)

49. [a] After the initial washing of general instruments, the instruments are placed in an ultrasonic cleaner, which removes debris that may have been missed.

After the initial washing of general instruments, the instruments are placed in an ultrasonic cleaner, which removes debris that may have been missed. (*page 161*)

50. [a] Ultrasonic cleaner

Dissimilar metals, such as copper, stainless steel, and brass, should not be combined in the ultrasonic cleaner. (*page 161*)

51. [c] Be lubricated with a water-soluble solution and then allowed to dry

Instruments that have been in the ultrasonic cleaner should be lubricated with a water-soluble solution and then allowed to dry. (*page 162*)

52. [a] (1), (2), and (3)

Box locks of instruments are opened for the sterilization cycle; heavy instruments should be placed in the bottom of the sterilizing tray; and delicate instruments are wrapped separately and placed on the top of the heavy instruments. Instrument sets should not exceed approximately 16 lb, and items with lumina should be flushed with distilled water when being prepared for steam sterilization. (*page 162*)

53. [d] Linen packs go on the top level of the sterilizer and metal on the bottom when running a mixed load.

Linen packages go on the top level of the sterilizer and metal on the bottom when running a mixed load. (*page 162*)

54. [b] It should not be placed near air vents or fans to avoid the possibility of condensation

After the sterilizer cart is removed from the autoclave, it should not be placed near air vents or fans to avoid the possibility of condensation. (*page 162*)

55. [b] When flashing metal instruments, the instruments are sterilized for 3 minutes at or above 270°F.

When flashing metal instruments, the instruments are sterilized for 3 minutes at or above 270°F. (*page 163*)

56. [c] Ethylene glycol

The combination of water and ethylene oxide forms ethylene glycol, a toxic substance. (*page 163*)

57. [a] Decrease ethylene oxide vapor build-up

After the ethylene oxide sterilization cycle is complete, the sterilizer door should be opened as soon as possible after completion of the sterilization cycle to decrease ethylene oxide vapor build-up. (*page 163*)

58. [b] Ethylene oxide can burn the skin

One should avoid touching ethylene oxide–sterilized items when transferring the items to the aerator because ethylene oxide can burn the skin. (*page 163*)

59. [a] Efficacy of the vacuum system of a prevacuum sterilizer

The Bowie-Dick test is carried out to determine the efficacy of the vacuum system of a prevacuum sterilizer. (*page 164*)

60. [d] (3) and (4)

Bacillus subtilis is used to test ethylene oxide sterilizers, and *Bacillus stearothermophilus* is used to test steam sterilizers. (*page 165*).

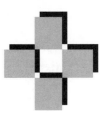

CHAPTER 11

Positioning the Patient

Positioning the patient describes activities done by the nurse to ensure that the patient is placed on the operative or invasive procedure bed in the best possible position to achieve maximum exposure of the operative site and to facilitate the performance of the procedure. The nurse must accomplish this while maintaining musculoskeletal and neurological safety, skin and tissue integrity, body alignment, and optimal physiological functioning of the respiratory and circulatory systems of the patient during the operative or invasive procedure. The questions for this chapter will help the reader assess his or her knowledge about

- Identifying the patient's risk for adverse outcomes related to positioning
- Selecting the appropriate supplies and equipment based on the patient's identified needs
- Preparing the bed
- Centering the patient on the bed
- Placing the patient's arms on armboards
- Using positioning devices according to the established practice recommendations and the manufacturer's recommendations
- Padding bony prominences
- Moving the anesthetized patient
- Documenting and communicating risk factors, nursing diagnoses, expected outcomes, the plan of care, interventions, and evaluation
- Placing the patient in the following positions: supine, Trendelenburg, reverse Trendelenburg, high and low lithotomy, lateral decubitus, prone, jackknife, and sitting

The reference used for this chapter is Phippen, M. L., & Wells, M. P. (1999). *Patient care during operative and invasive procedures.* Philadelphia: W. B. Saunders, pp. 167–182.

Questions

1. The nurse must possess various knowledge and skills to successfully fulfill his or her duties when positioning a surgical patient. These are best summarized as:

   a. Problem solving, communication and assessment skills, and knowledge of anatomy and anesthesia

   b. Problem solving and assessment skills, and knowledge of the operating room (OR) bed, surgical procedure, and potential complications

   c. Problem solving, communication, and assessment skills, and knowledge of the operation of the OR bed and the surgical procedure

   d. Problem solving and documentation skills and knowledge of the surgical procedure, functioning of the OR bed, and positioning devices

2. *Surgical positioning does not physically compromise or cause injury to the patient* is an example of an outcome standard associated with positioning of the surgical patient. Which of the following criteria best measures achievement of this outcome standard?

   a. The patient does not show evidence of skin breakdown related to positioning.

   b. The patient shows no evidence of ineffective breathing patterns during the postprocedure period.

   c. The patient does not show evidence of injury related to position, such as signs of difficulty in ambulation.

d. The patient shows no evidence of altered tissue perfusion related to positioning, such as blood pressure changes.

3. The nurse is responsible for assessing the patient to determine the presence of risk factors for potential bodily injury related to positioning. What factors place the patient at risk for injury related to positioning?

a. Muscle weakness, paralysis, incoordination, sensory deterioration, and infection

b. Trauma, age, inadequate staff, shortage of equipment, and a hazardous environment

c. Impaired judgment, disorientation, incoordination, anesthesia, and inattentive staff

d. Paralysis, previous accidental trauma, sensory deterioration, impaired judgment, and a hazardous environment

4. When the patient's arms are being positioned on armboards:

a. The armboards should be the same height as the bed pads

b. The armboards should be at a 95-degree angle to the body

c. The palms should be supinated (facing upward)

d. The palms should be elevated

5. When the patient's arms are being positioned at his or her side:

a. The arms should be turned away from the patient's sides

b. The arms should be secured with the safety strap

c. The elbows should be flexed

d. The fingers should be clear of the OR bed breaks

6. Shearing is a potential injury factor related to surgical positioning. In which of the following positions is the potential for shearing injury to tissues greatest?

a. Supine

b. Reverse Trendelenburg

c. Lateral decubitus

d. Prone

7. When the patient is being positioned on the OR bed in the supine position:

a. The safety strap should be placed 2 inches below the knees

b. The safety strap should be secured so that a hand cannot be inserted under it

c. The head, spine, and legs should be in alignment

d. The patient's legs should be slightly flexed and crossed

8. The nurse should assess the surgical patient for risk factors related to impaired skin integrity. What factors place the patient at risk for impaired skin integrity?

a. Shearing forces, physical immobilization, and edema

b. Pressure on the nervous system, emaciation, and pooling of preparation solutions

c. Inattentive staff leaning on patient, prolonged pressure on bony prominences, and obesity

d. All of the above

9. The nurse should assess the patient for risk factors related to ineffective breathing patterns. Which factor can contribute to the patient's experiencing respirations inadequate to maintain sufficient oxygen supply for cellular requirements?

a. Shearing forces or change in skin turgor

b. Obesity or emaciation

c. Pregnancy or hormonal disorders

d. Existing neuromuscular or musculoskeletal impairment

10. The nurse should assess the surgical patient for risk factors related to altered tissue perfusion. All of the following factors contribute to altered tissue perfusion, except:

a. Excessive abduction of the arms on armboards

b. Excessive adduction of the arms on armboards

c. Compression of extremities against positioning devices

d. Inattentive staff leaning on the patient

11. The nurse should be able to recognize evidence of altered tissue perfusion related to surgical positioning. Which condition indicates altered tissue perfusion?

a. Flushing of the extremity

b. Increased arterial pulsation

c. Edema of the extremities

d. Nerve damage

12. The nurse needs to communicate with the patient and other members of the surgical team. Which statement concerning communication is not correct?

a. Family members should be consulted concerning potential positioning problems that the patient may experience.

b. The patient should be informed of the positioning procedure during teaching.

c. Intraoperative needs of the patient should be communicated to other members of the surgical team.

d. The postprocedure evaluation should be communicated to other members of the surgical team.

13. The nurse is responsible for preparing the OR bed before transferring the pa-

tient. Which statement concerning the preparation of the OR bed is correct?

a. The bed should be clean, free from hazards, and unlocked to allow for movement.

b. All required positioning devices should be attached to the bed before the patient is transferred.

c. A padded foot extension should be attached if the patient's feet will extend beyond the end of the bed.

d. Pads should be graduated in height to enhance venous return.

14. The nurse is responsible for coordinating the moving of an anesthetized patient. Which statement concerning the movement of an anesthetized patient is correct?

a. Inform the anesthetist when moving or repositioning the anesthetized patient.

b. Move the patient quickly, with firm, steady motions.

c. Reassess the patient for body alignment and tissue integrity after draping.

d. Move the patient only if adequate personnel to assist are available.

15. The most frequently used position for patients undergoing surgical procedures is the supine position. This is also known as the:

a. Ventral recumbent

b. Dorsal recumbent

c. Parasagittal transverse

d. Caudal inferior

16. Which statement best describes a patient in the supine position?

a. On the back, with the arms at the sides

b. On the back, with the head elevated

c. On the back, with the arms flexed

d. On the back, with legs flexed

17. Which of the following factors should be taken into consideration when determining the minimal number of staff needed to position the patient?

    a. The proposed position

    b. The size of the patient

    c. The safety of the operative team

    d. All of the above

18. Potential adverse reactions to the supine position include:

    a. Position-induced hypertension

    b. Increased diaphragmatic excursion

    c. Restriction of posterolateral chest movement

    d. Increased mean arterial pressure

19. Which list of supplies best describes the basic supplies that should be available to position the patient in the supine position?

    a. Pillow, armboards, and padded footboards

    b. Headrest, arm restraint, and safety strap

    c. Pillow, padding, and safety strap

    d. Headrest, armboard, and pelvic wedge

20. Which of the following patients would be at greatest risk for potential complications from the supine position?

    a. Pregnant patient

    b. Geriatric patient

    c. Immunosuppressed patient

    d. Diabetic patient

21. After transfer to the OR bed, the patient should be assessed to ensure that:

    a. The head, neck, and legs are in proper alignment

b. The legs are crossed and secured with safety strap

c. The legs are flexed with safety strap over the knees

d. A pillow is placed between the knees and the feet are padded

22. The nurse should be aware of the potential for injury to which body structures?

    a. Scalp, lumbar plexus, occiput, and hips

    b. Skin over bony prominences, brachial plexus, sacrum, and popliteal artery

    c. Common peroneal nerve, scapulae, shoulders, and feet

    d. Ears, diaphragm, ulnar nerve, and superior vena cava

23. In the supine position, padding should be placed:

    a. Under the neck

    b. Under the axilla

    c. Under the upper lumbar area

    d. Under the knees

24. A small pelvic wedge should be placed under the right side for pregnant or obese patients to:

    a. Improve diaphragmatic excursion

    b. Prevent joint injury

    c. Relieve sacral pressure

    d. Relieve pressure on the inferior vena cava

25. Potential adverse reactions related to the Trendelenburg position include:

    a. Hypertension and increased cardiac output

    b. Cerebral hypoxia due to decreased venous pressure

    c. Venous thrombosis and stagnation

    d. Lung compression by the abdominal contents

26. Body structures at risk for injury in the Trendelenburg position include:

   a. Scalp, brachial plexus, occiput, and calf muscles

   b. Occiput, cervical plexus, sacrum, and hips

   c. Ears, sacral plexus, calcaneus, and inferior vena cava

   d. Sacrum, common peroneal nerve, diaphragm, and brachial artery

27. Which supplies should be available to position the patient in the Trendelenburg position?

   a. Pillow, armboard, and safety strap

   b. Headrest, armboard, and shoulder braces

   c. Pillow, safety strap, and pelvic wedge

   d. Armboards, padding, and shoulder braces

28. The Trendelenburg position is used for what types of surgical procedures?

   a. Thoracic procedures

   b. Procedures on organs in the pelvic cavity

   c. Procedures on facial structures

   d. Procedures on the extremities

29. The reverse Trendelenburg position is used for what type of surgical procedures?

   a. Thoracic procedures

   b. Procedures on organs in the pelvic cavity

   c. Procedures of the head and neck

   d. Extremity procedures

30. When positioning the patient in the reverse Trendelenburg position, the nurse should be alert to what potential adverse effect?

   a. Increased pressure on the diaphragm

   b. Venous pooling in the legs

   c. Popliteal nerve damage

   d. Hypotension

31. Which body structures are at risk for injury in the reverse Trendelenburg position?

   a. Scalp, brachial plexus, and calcaneus

   b. Ears, elbows, and saphenous vein

   c. Skin over bony prominences, sacrum, and ankles

   d. Occiput, sacral plexus, and popliteal artery

32. What supplies should be available to safely position the patient in the reverse Trendelenburg position?

   a. Armboards, padding, and shoulder braces

   b. Armboards, padded knee rest, and safety strap

   c. Armboards, pillow, and padded footboard

   d. Headrest, safety strap, and axillary roll

33. The lithotomy position, high or low, is used for what types of surgical procedures?

   a. Procedures on the extremities

   b. Procedures requiring a vaginal or perineal approach

   c. Thoracic procedures

   d. Venous procedures

34. The nurse should be aware of what potential adverse effect of positioning in the lithotomy position?

   a. Venous pooling in the legs

b. Venous compression of nervous structures

c. Diaphragmatic pressure on abdominal contents

d. Hypotension when the legs are lowered

35. What is the least number of personnel needed to safely position the patient in the lithotomy position?

a. One

b. Two

c. Three

d. Four

36. Which body structures are at risk for injury in the lithotomy position?

a. Skin over bony prominences, lumbar plexus, and hips

b. Occiput, sternum, and saphenous vein

c. Scalp, sacrum, and common peroneal nerve

d. Brachial plexus, spinous processes, and ankles

37. When taking a patient out of the lithotomy position, the nurse should be careful to:

a. Slowly lower the extended legs one at a time

b. Slowly lower the extended legs together

c. Avoid excessive adduction of the legs while they are being lowered

d. Lower the legs in flexed position, then extend

38. What supplies and equipment should the nurse have available to safely position the patient in the lithotomy position?

a. Pillow, safety strap, stirrups, and holders

b. Headrest, armboards, and protective leg covers

c. Pillow, safety strap, and padded footboard

d. Headrest, armboards, and sacral support

39. Important nursing considerations the nurse should be aware of when positioning the patient in lithotomy include:

a. Attach the stirrup holders to the OR bed below the knee break

b. Slowly flex the legs, internally rotate them, and place them in stirrups

c. Transfer the patient to the OR bed with the hips at the knee break

d. Ensure that stirrups are at the appropriate height and level

40. When removing the patient from the lithotomy position, the nurse should:

a. Place the head section and pad back on the head of the OR bed

b. Check that the fingers are not extending beyond the OR bed break

c. Lower the legs slowly, one at a time

d. Elevate the leg section beyond the vertical position

41. Which of the following is a modification of the supine position?

a. Prone position

b. Reverse Trendelenburg position

c. Jackknife position

d. All of the above

42. The lateral decubitus position is used for what types of surgery?

a. Plastic, gynecological, or hip procedures

b. Thoracic, neurological, or plastic procedures

c. Thoracic, renal, or hip procedures

d. Renal, genitourinary, or gynecological procedures

43. What is the least number of personnel needed to safely position the patient in the lateral decubitus position?

a. Two

b. Three

c. Four

d. Five

44. One potential adverse effect of the lateral decubitus position that the nurse should be alert to is:

a. Hypotension, more pronounced in the left lateral position

b. Injury to the elevated brachial plexus

c. Injury to the inferior vena cava

d. Interference with cardiac function due to a shift in heart position

45. The body structures at risk for injury in the lateral decubitus position are:

a. Ears, sciatic nerve, zygomatic arch, and diaphragm

b. Scalp, brachial plexus, hips, and popliteal artery

c. Eyelids, common peroneal nerve, clavicle, and abdominal aorta

d. Nose, suprascapular nerve, neck, and genitalia

46. An important aspect of communication that the nurse should be aware of is that:

a. All assistants understand their role in positioning the patient

b. Preprocedure medications are communicated to all personnel

c. Time of positioning the patient is communicated to anesthesia personnel

d. The surgeon communicates when the patient is ready to be positioned

47. Which member of the surgical team initiates movement of the patient?

a. Circulating nurse

b. Surgeon

c. Anesthetist

d. Assistants

48. The proper placement of personnel to safely move the patient into the lateral decubitus position is:

a. One person on each side and one at the patient's feet

b. Two people on the side that will be up, two on the opposite side, and one at the foot

c. Two people on the side that will be down, one on the opposite side, and one at the foot

d. Two people on each side of the patient

49. What should the nurse have available to safely position the patient in the lateral decubitus position?

a. Pillows, padding, and special positioning devices

b. Headrest, pillow, and chest rolls

c. Pillows, beanbag, and safety strap

d. Headrest, shoulder support, and safety strap

50. After the patient is moved into position:

a. A roll should be placed below the axilla

b. The upside leg should be flexed at the knee

c. A roll should be placed under the thorax

d. A pillow or padding should be placed under the legs

51. After positioning the patient, the nurse should ensure that:

    a. The axillary roll in is the axilla

    b. The genitals and breasts are free of pressure

    c. Both legs are padded and flexed

    d. The safety strap is secured below the knees

52. The prone position is also known as the:

    a. Caudal decubitus position

    b. Dorsal recumbent position

    c. Reverse supine position

    d. Ventral decubitus position

53. The prone position is used for what types of surgical procedures?

    a. Genitourinary and renal procedures

    b. Back and rectal procedures

    c. Thoracic and renal procedures

    d. Hip and lower extremity procedures

54. Body structures at risk for injury in the prone position include:

    a. Carotid artery, dorsal area of feet, and sciatic nerve

    b. Popliteal artery, hips, and diaphragm

    c. Abdominal aorta, spine, and knees

    d. Carotid artery, neck muscles, and brachial plexus

55. What is the least number of personnel needed to safely position the patient in the prone position?

    a. Two

    b. Three

    c. Four

    d. Five

56. The nurse should be alert to what potential adverse effect when the patient is positioned in the prone position?

    a. Pressure on the inferior vena cava, resulting in hypotension

    b. Excessive intraoperative bleeding

    c. Injury to nerves and tendons of the dorsa of the feet

    d. All of the above

57. What supplies should the nurse have available to safely position the patient in the prone position?

    a. Pillows, axillary roll, and supporting frame

    b. Headrest, armboards, and safety strap

    c. Headrest, chest rolls, and safety strap

    d. Pillows, padding, and padded knee rest

58. When moving the patient, the nurse should make sure that:

    a. The arms are over the patient's head

    b. The arms are at the patient's sides

    c. Personnel are placed at each side and at the foot of the OR bed

    d. The patient is moved by the chest and legs

59. After turning the patient, the nurse should ensure that:

    a. The chest rolls extend from the clavicle to the iliac crest

    b. The chest rolls extend from the acromioclavicular joint to the hips

    c. The breasts are displaced laterally to prevent injury

    d. The safety strap is secured 2 inches below the knees

60. Pressure areas that should be checked after positioning include:

    a. The soles of the feet

    b. The popliteal space

    c. The genitalia

    d. The shoulders

61. The jackknife position is also known as the:

    a. Modified prone position

    b. Kraske position

    c. Fowler position

    d. Sims position

62. The jackknife position is used for what type of surgical procedures?

    a. Gluteal and anorectal procedures

    b. Renal and genitourinary procedures

    c. Back and hip procedures

    d. Extremity and gynecological procedures

63. What is the least number of personnel needed to safely position the patient in the jackknife position?

    a. Two

    b. Three

    c. Four

    d. Five

64. What structures are at risk for injury when the patient is in the jackknife position?

    a. Ears, scapula, dorsal area of the foot

    b. Eyelids, common peroneal nerve, hips

    c. Brachial plexus, carotid artery, genitalia

    d. Cornea, diaphragm, popliteal artery

65. The nurse needs to be aware that the potential adverse effects of positioning in the jackknife position are the same as the potential adverse effects of the:

    a. Lithotomy position

    b. Lateral decubitus position

    c. Sitting position

    d. Prone position

66. What supplies should the nurse have available to safely position the patient in the jackknife position?

    a. Headrest, arm restraints, safety strap

    b. Pillows, chest rolls, safety strap

    c. Headrest, supporting frame, armboards

    d. Pillows, padding, back brace

67. When positioning the patient in the Kraske position, the nurse should ensure that:

    a. The patient's hips are positioned over the OR bed break

    b. The arms are at a 90-degree angle or less

    c. The safety strap is secure and 2 inches below the knees

    d. The soles of the feet are padded to prevent pressure

68. The sitting position is used for which type of surgical procedures?

    a. Neurosurgical procedures

    b. Plastic procedures

    c. Orthopedic procedures

    d. Otorhinolaryngeal procedures

69. What is the least number of personnel needed to safely position the patient in the sitting position?

    a. One

    b. Two

    c. Three

    d. Four

70. What body structures are at risk for injury when the patient is positioned in the sitting position?

    a. Cervical spine, abdominal aorta, popliteal artery

b. Eyelids, sacrum, superficial temporal artery

c. Sciatic nerve, scapula, saphenous vein

d. Superior vena cava, common peroneal nerve, hips

71. The potential adverse effects of the sitting position to which the nurse needs to be alert include:

a. Intraoperative hypotension

b. Venous air embolism

c. Pressure on the Achilles tendon

d. All of the above

72. What supplies should the nurse have available to safely position the patient in the sitting position?

a. Head holder, padded footboard, safety strap

b. Chest rolls, padding, padded footboard

c. Head holder, armboards, safety strap

d. Headrest, pillows, padding

73. Before transferring the patient, the nurse should:

a. Attach the padded footrest to the OR bed

b. Apply compression stockings to both legs

c. Assess the genitals for pressure

d. Secure the skull clamp to the holder

74. The intraoperative nursing record should include:

a. Position

b. Safety and security measures

c. Use and location of positioning devices

d. All of the above

◆ Answers

1. [c] Problem solving, communication, assessment skills, and knowledge of the operation of the OR bed and the surgical procedure

To safely position a surgical patient, the nurse should possess skill in problem solving, communication, and assessment, as well as knowledge of operation of the OR bed and surgical procedure. (*page 167*)

2. [a] The patient does not show evidence of skin breakdown related to positioning

According to the Association of Operating Room Nurses Outcome Standards, the patient should not show evidence of skin breakdown, ineffective breathing patterns, altered skin perfusion, or postprocedure pain related to positioning. (*page 168*)

3. [d] Paralysis, previous accidental trauma, sensory deterioration, impaired judgment, and a hazardous environment

Factors that place the patient at risk for injury include disorientation, impaired judgment, muscle weakness, paralysis, incoordination, sensory/perceptual deterioration, existing or previous trauma, lack of safety precautions attributed to staff, shortage of equipment, and a hazardous environment. (*page 169*)

4. [a] The armboards should be the same height as the bed pads

Armboards should be positioned at less than a 90-degree angle to the patient's body. The armboards and table should be the same height. Each arm is secured with a safety strap. (*page 168*)

5. [d] The fingers should be clear of the OR bed breaks

The elbows must be checked to ensure that they are not flexed or resting on the metal edge of the bed. The fingers must be clear of the OR bed breaks and other possible hazards. (*page 168*)

6. [b] Reverse Trendelenburg

The reverse Trendelenburg position places the patient at greatest danger for injury from shearing forces if the patient slides toward the foot of the bed. (*page 174*)

7. [c] The head, spine, and legs should be in alignment

After transfer from the gurney, the patient's head, spine, and legs should be checked for proper alignment. The legs should not be crossed and should remain slightly apart. (*page 168*)

8. [d] All of the above

Factors that place the patient at risk for impaired skin integrity include prolonged pressure, shearing forces, pressure on peripheral nerves or blood vessels, physical immobilization of longer than 90 minutes, staff leaning on patient, obesity or emaciation, change in skin turgor, edema, and pooling of prep solutions. (*page 169*)

9. [d] Existing neuromuscular or musculoskeletal impairment

Factors that place the patient at risk for ineffective breathing patterns include obesity, staff leaning on the patient, existing neuromuscular or musculoskeletal impairment, and pregnancy. (*page 169*)

10. [b] Excessive adduction of the arms on armboards

Factors that place the patient at risk for altered tissue perfusion include compression of extremities against positioning devices or operative bed accessories, and pregnancy. (*page 169*)

11. [c] Edema of the extremities

Altered tissue perfusion may be evidenced by cold extremities, diminished pulses, blood pressure changes in extremities, edema, or discoloration in the extremities. (*page 169*)

12. [a] Family members should be consulted concerning potential positioning problems that the patient may experience.

Communication with the patient and members of the operative or invasive procedure team is essential. The nurse should inform the patient of the positioning procedure during the patient teaching session. Family members may not be aware of potential positioning problems that the patient may experience but are aware of specific patient requirements. (*page 172*)

13. [c] A padded foot extension should be attached if the patient's feet will extend beyond the end of the bed.

All portions of the patient's body should be supported. After transfer from the gurney, the patient's head, neck, spine, and legs should be checked for proper alignment. (*page 173*)

14. [d] Move the patient with adequate personnel to assist only.

The patient should not be moved unless adequate assistance is available. (*page 168*)

15. [b] Dorsal recumbent

The supine position is also known as the dorsal recumbent position. This is the most frequently used position for patients undergoing an operative procedure. (*page 172*)

16. [a] On the back, with the arms at the sides

In the supine position, the patient is placed on his or her back with the legs extended and the arms resting on armboards or at the sides. This position is routinely used in abdominal, thoracic, vascular, and orthopedic procedures. (*page 172*)

17. [d] All of the above

The nurse is the minimum nursing staff needed to position the patient. However, staffing requirements should be based on the need to provide safe patient care without jeopardizing the safety of the operative team. (*page 172*)

18. [c] Restriction of posterolateral chest movement

Potential adverse effects of positioning in the supine position include hypotension, venous pooling in the legs, decreased diaphragmatic excursion, restriction of posterolateral chest movement, and decreased mean arterial pressure, heart rate, and peripheral resistance. (*page 172*)

19. [c] Pillow, padding, and safety strap

The routine supplies needed for placing the patient in the supine position are armboards, arm restraints, pillow or headrest, padding, and a safety strap. (*page 173*)

20. [a] Pregnant patient

Pregnant or obese patients in the supine position are at danger for pressure on the vena cava. A small pelvic wedge placed under the right side of the patient relieves pressure on the vena cava. (*page 173*)

21. [a] The head, neck, and legs are in proper alignment

The nurse should ensure that the patient's head, neck, and legs are in proper alignment and that the legs are not crossed and remain slightly apart. (*page 168*)

22. [b] Skin over bony prominences, brachial plexus, sacrum, and popliteal artery

Structures at risk for injury in the supine position include the skin over bony prominences, brachial plexus sacrum, and popliteal artery. (*page 170*)

23. [d] Under the knees

In the supine position, padding should be placed under the patient's head, lower lumbar area, knees, and heels. (*page 173*)

24. [d] Relieve pressure on the inferior vena cava

For pregnant or obese patients, a small pelvic wedge is placed under the right side to relieve pressure on the inferior vena cava. (*page 173*)

25. [d] Lung compression by the abdominal contents

Potential adverse effects in the Trendelenburg position include hypotension, air embo-

lism, retinal detachment or cerebral edema, venous thrombosis, occlusion of superficial veins, atelectasis, or nerve injury. (*page 173*)

26. [a] Scalp, brachial plexus, occiput, and calf muscles

Body structures at risk for injury in the Trendelenburg position include the scalp, brachial plexus, occiput, and calf muscles. (*page 170*)

27. [a] Pillow, armboard, and safety strap

The routine supplies needed for placing the patient in the Trendelenburg position include armboards, arm restraints, a pillow or headrest, padding, and a safety strap. (*page 173*)

28. [b] Procedures on organs in the pelvic cavity

The Trendelenburg position causes the abdominal organs to move out of the pelvis, improving visualization of the pelvic organs. (*page 173*)

29. [c] Procedures of the head and neck

The reverse Trendelenburg position is used for procedures of the head and neck. (*page 174*)

30. [b] Venous pooling in the legs

Potential adverse effects of the reverse Trendelenburg position include venous pooling in legs, radial median or ulnar nerve damage, and impaired tissue integrity from shearing forces. (*page 174*)

31. [a] Scalp, brachial plexus, and calcaneus

Body structures at risk for injury in the reverse Trendelenburg position include the scalp, brachial plexus, and calcaneus. (*page 170*)

32. [c] Armboards, pillows, and padded footboard

The routine supplies needed to place the patient in the reverse Trendelenburg position are armboards, arm restraints, a padded footboard, padding, and a safety strap. (*page 174*)

33. [b] Procedures requiring a vaginal or perineal approach

The lithotomy position is used for procedures requiring a vaginal or perineal approach. (*page 174*)

34. [d] Hypotension when the legs are lowered

Potential adverse effects of the lithotomy position include venous pooling, vein compression in the groin and legs, increased intra-abdominal pressure, severe hypotension, injury to the obturator and femoral nerves, injury to the saphenous and common peroneal nerves, and hip and brachial plexus injury. (*page 175*)

35. [b] Two

The nurse and an assistant are the minimal nursing staff needed to position the patient in lithotomy position. (*page 175*)

36. [c] Scalp, sacrum, and common peroneal nerve

Body structures at risk for injury in the lithotomy position include the scalp, sacrum, and common peroneal nerve. (*page 170*)

37. [b] Slowly lower the extended legs together

Severe hypotension due to blood's draining from the torso into the legs may result if legs are lowered too quickly. (*page 176*)

38. [a] Pillow, safety strap, stirrups and holders

The routine supplies needed for placing the patient in lithotomy position are armboards, arm restraints, a pillow or headrest, padding, a safety strap, protective leg coverings, stirrups, and stirrup holders. (*page 176*)

39. [d] Ensure that stirrups are at the appropriate height and level

The nurse should adjust the stirrups, ensuring that they are at the appropriate height and level and are secure. (*page 175*)

40. [b] Check that the fingers are not extending beyond the OR bed break

The nurse should check that the patient's hands and fingers are not extending beyond the OR bed break. (*page 176*)

41. [b] Reverse Trendelenburg position

The reverse Trendelenburg position is a modification of the supine position. (*page 174*)

42. [c] Thoracic, renal, or hip procedures

The lateral decubitus position is used for thoracic, renal, and orthopedic (hip) procedures. (*page 177*)

43. [d] Five

The nurse and four assistants are the minimum nursing staff needed to position the patient in the lateral decubitus position. (*page 177*)

44. [d] Interference with cardiac function due to a shift in heart position

Potential adverse effects in the lateral decubitus position include injury to the dependent brachial plexus; injury to the median, radial, ulnar and peroneal nerves; pressure sore development over dependent greater trochanter of the femur; interference with cardiac action due to shift in cardiac position; drop in arterial pressure. (*page 178*)

45. [a] Ears, sciatic nerve, zygomatic arch, and diaphragm

Body structures at risk for injury in the lateral decubitus position include the ears, sciatic nerve, zygomatic arch, and diaphragm. (*page 170*)

46. [a] All assistants understand their role in positioning the patient

It is important the nurse ensures that all assistants understand their individual roles in positioning the patient. (*page 178*)

47. [c] Anesthetist

The anesthetist controls the head and neck and initiates the movement of the patient during positioning. (*page 178*)

48. [b] Two people on the side that will be up, two on the opposite side, and one at the foot

Proper placement of personnel for positioning the patient in the lateral decubitus position has the nurse and one assistant opposite the side that will be down, two assistants to the side that will be down, and one assistant at the foot. (*page 178*)

49. [c] Pillows, beanbag, and safety strap

The routine supplies needed to position the patient in the lateral decubitus position are pillows, a headrest, padding, armboards, a safety strap, a beanbag, and other special positioning equipment. (*page 177*)

50. [a] A roll should be placed below the axilla

After the patient is moved into position, a rolled towel or other type of padding (axillary roll) should be placed under the patient below the axilla, not in the axilla. (*page 178*)

51. [b] The genitals and breasts are free of pressure

After positioning the patient, the nurse should ensure that the genitals and breasts are free of pressure. (*page 178*)

52. [d] Ventral decubitus position

The prone position is also known as the ventral recumbent or ventral decubitus position. (*page 178*)

53. [b] Back and rectal procedures

The prone position is used for procedures of the cervical spine, back, rectal area, and lower extremities. (*page 178*)

54. [d] Carotid artery, neck muscles, and brachial plexus

Body structures at risk for injury in the prone position include the carotid artery, neck muscles, and brachial plexus. (*page 170*)

55. [d] Five

The nurse and four assistants are the minimal nursing staff needed to position the patient in the prone position. (*page 178*)

56. [d] All of the above

Potential adverse effects in the prone position include pressure on the vena cava, causing hypotension, excessive blood loss from veins of the vertebral column, and injury to the brachial plexus, lateral femoral cutaneous, facial, and ulnar nerves, tendons and nerves of the dorsa of the feet, and the genitalia and breasts. (*page 179*)

57. [c] Headrest, chest rolls, and safety strap

The routine supplies needed to position the patient in the prone position are pillows, headrest, chest rolls or a supporting frame, padding, armboards, arm restraints, and a safety strap. (*page 178*)

58. [b] The arms are at the patient's sides

The nurse should ensure that the patient's arms are at his or her sides. (*page 179*)

59. [a] The chest rolls extend from the clavicle to the iliac crest

The nurse should ensure that chest rolls extend from the acromioclavicular joint to the iliac crest and do not impinge on the chest expansion. (*page 179*)

60. [c] The genitalia

After positioning, the nurse should ensure that there is no pressure on the genitals. (*page 179*)

61. [b] Kraske position

The jackknife position is also known as the Kraske position. (*page 179*)

62. [a] Gluteal and anorectal procedures

The jackknife position is used for gluteal and anorectal procedures. (*page 179*)

63. [d] Five

The nurse and four assistants are the minimal nursing staff needed to position the patient in the jackknife position. (*page 179*)

64. [c] Brachial plexus, carotid artery, genitalia

Body structures at risk for injury in the jackknife position include the brachial plexus, carotid artery, and genitalia. (*page 170*)

65. [d] Prone position

The potential adverse effects of the jackknife position are the same as those of the prone position. (*page 179*)

66. [b] Pillows, chest rolls, and safety strap

The routine supplies needed to place the patient in the jackknife position are pillows, a headrest, chest rolls or a supporting frame, padding, armboards, arm restraints, and a safety strap. (*page 180*)

67. [a] The patient's hips are positioned over the OR bed break

The nurse should ensure that the patient's hips are over the OR bed break. (*page 180*)

68. [a] Neurosurgical procedures

The sitting position is used for neurosurgical procedures. (*page 180*)

69. [a] One

The nurse is the minimal nursing staff needed to position the patient in the sitting position. (*page 180*)

70. [c] Sciatic nerve, scapula, saphenous vein

Body structures at risk for injury in the sitting position include the sciatic nerve, the scapula, and the saphenous vein. (*page 170*)

71. [d] All of the above

Potential adverse effects in the sitting position include hypotension, venous pooling in the legs, venous air embolism, pressure on the ischial tuberosity, injury to the sciatic nerve, and footdrop due to pressure on the Achilles tendon. (*page 180*)

72. [a] Head holder, padded footboard, safety strap

The routine supplies needed to position the patient in the sitting position include armboards, arm restraints, a head holder, padding, a padded footboard, and a safety strap. (*page 180*)

73. [b] Apply compression stockings to both legs

Before placing the patient in the sitting position, the nurse should wrap both of the patient's legs to the groin with elastic bandages or compression stockings. (*page 181*)

74. [d] All of the above

The intraoperative nursing record should include the position, safety, and security measures and the use and location of positioning devices. (*page 172*)

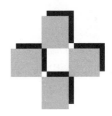

CHAPTER 12

Handling Cultures and Specimens

Handling cultures and specimens describes patient care activities performed by the nurse and other members of the patient care team to collect, process, store, preserve, and transport operative and invasive procedure cultures and tissue specimens. The questions for this chapter will help the reader assess his or her knowledge about

- Identifying legal implications of handling cultures and specimens
- Discussing infection control implications of handling cultures and specimens
- Identifying safe precautions for handling formalin
- Identifying the patient's risk for adverse outcomes related to handling cultures and specimens
- Providing supplies and equipment needed for the collection of cultures and specimens
- Labeling cultures and specimens
- Completing laboratory requisition slips
- Documenting the collection of cultures and specimens on the patient's operative record
- Establishing chain of custody for cultures and tissue specimens
- Collecting and preparing cultures for examination
- Collecting and preparing tissue for examination
- Storing, preserving, and maintaining tissue
- Directing the transfer of cultures and specimens to the laboratory
- Communicating pathology reports to the physician

The reference used for this chapter is Phippen, M.L., & Wells, M.P. (1999). *Patient care during operative and invasive procedures.* Philadelphia: W. B. Saunders, pp. 183–190.

✚ Questions

1. All cultures and specimens are:

   a. Sterile

   b. Fixed with formalin

   c. Potentially infectious

   d. The property of the patient

2. Because formalin is a hazardous material by federal law, the manufacturer must supply:

   a. Fire extinguishers

   b. Material safety data sheets (MSDSs)

   c. Personal protective equipment

   d. Inservices to the hospital

3. When should the nurse gather the supplies and equipment for cultures and specimens?

   a. When a request from the surgeon has been made to send a specimen

   b. After the patient has been intubated

   c. Before the patient is transferred to the operating room bed

   d. Never; the nursing assistant should gather supplies

4. To ensure continuity of care for the patient, the nurse must:

   a. Properly label cultures and specimens

   b. Accept responsibility for errors

   c. Wear sterile gloves

d. Disinfect the exterior of the specimen cup

5. To ensure an appropriate diagnosis from the pathology department, the nurse should:

a. Repeat the name of the test to the scrub nurse

b. Walk the specimen to the laboratory

c. Delegate the task of collecting the specimen to the nursing assistant

d. Properly label the specimen

6. In high concentrations, formalin vapors may cause:

a. Sore throats

b. Coughing

c. Shortness of breath

d. Death

7. In the event of a formalin spill, one should:

a. Pull the fire alarm

b. Ventilate the area

c. Alert the emergency department to expect patients

d. Pour a solution of sodium bicarbonate over the spill area

8. The purpose of the laboratory slip is to:

a. Identify the type of study requested

b. Prevent lost specimens

c. Identify the person transporting the specimen

d. Inform the nurse on how to collect the specimen

9. What mechanism is used to ensure accountability for cultures and tissue specimens?

a. Log book

b. Chain of custody

c. Labeling of specimens

d. Completing laboratory slips

10. What is used to track the specimen from the surgical suite to the pathology department?

a. Intraoperative record

b. Labels

c. Log book

d. Laboratory slips

11. The purpose of the culture is to:

a. Start the correct treatment

b. Document the surgical intervention

c. Prevent the spread of contamination in the operating room

d. Identify the pathogen causing the infection

12. Microorganisms that require the presence of oxygen for survival are called:

a. Aerobic bacteria

b. Anaerobic bacteria

c. Microaerophilic bacteria

d. Fungi

13. Microorganisms that grow in the absence of oxygen are categorized as:

a. Aerobic bacteria

b. Anaerobic bacteria

c. Viruses

d. Fungi

14. How many specimens can be placed in each container?

a. One

b. Two

c. Four

d. Six

15. An example of a gram-negative bacillus is:

    a. *Streptococcus*

    b. *Histoplasma capsulatum*

    c. *Salmonella*

    d. *Mycobacterium tuberculosis*

16. What would the nurse use to decontaminate the exterior of the culture tube?

    a. Gluteraldehyde

    b. 70% ethyl alcohol

    c. Soap and water

    d. 1 : 10 dilution of household bleach

17. A tuberculocidal hospital disinfectant is:

    a. Ethylene oxide gas

    b. 70% alcohol

    c. Gluteraldehyde

    d. 1 : 10 dilution of household bleach

18. The test done to assist in the classification of the genus of bacteria is known as:

    a. Gram stain

    b. Acid-fast cultures

    c. Fungal smears

    d. Aerobic cultures

19. The container used to collect a specimen for a Gram stain is:

    a. A nonsterile container

    b. An aerobic culture tube

    c. A syringe with all the air removed

    d. A glass slide

20. Gram-negative bacteria appear:

    a. Yellow

    b. Purple

    c. Blue

    d. Pink

21. Gram-positive bacteria retain the color:

    a. Red

    b. Pink

    c. Blue

    d. Yellow

22. The minimal amount of spinal fluid needed for an acid-fast culture and smear is:

    a. 2.0 mL

    b. 1.5 mL

    c. 1.0 mL

    d. 0.5 mL

23. The test done to assist in the diagnosis of tuberculosis is:

    a. A Gram stain

    b. An acid-fast culture

    c. A spinal tap

    d. An anaerobic culture

24. Fluid specimens:

    a. Must be hand carried to the laboratory

    b. Should be in anaerobic culture tubes

    c. Should not be shaken

    d. Should be shaken

25. Fluid specimens should not be shaken because this:

    a. Prevents correct Gram staining

    b. Can seed the cancer cell

    c. Makes it more difficult to fix a permanent specimen

    d. May rupture the cell

26. Tissue, particularly that sent for frozen specimens, should remain:

    a. In a near-natural state

    b. In a dry, sterile specimen container

c. In the operating room until the end of the procedure

d. On the sterile field until the pathologist is able to collect the specimen

27. All tissue or objects removed from the patient are sent to the laboratory as permanent specimens. Exceptions to this guideline are dictated by:

a. Physicians in charge of the case

b. Hospital policy

c. Insurance coverage of the patient

d. Supervisors of the pathology department

28. To prevent inadvertent discarding of the specimen during cleanup after the procedure, the specimen should be:

a. Labeled immediately

b. Placed in the upper right-hand corner of the back table

c. Handed off the sterile field as soon as possible

d. Placed in a large stainless steel basin

29. Why are bladder or gallstones sent to the laboratory in a dry container?

a. It prevents decomposition.

b. Specimens need to arrive in a near-natural state.

c. Pathologists prefer this technique.

d. It prevents formation of crystals.

30. If a specimen is difficult to see because of size, it should be placed on a:

a. Glass slide

b. Material that provides contrast

c. Petri dish

d. Gentian violet–soaked 4 × 4 inch pad

31. The frozen section examination provides the surgeon with a:

a. Guideline for antibiotic therapy

b. Diagnosis for tuberculosis

c. Quick preliminary diagnosis

d. Microscopic examination of smears and cultures

32. Frozen sections are analyzed to:

a. Guide antibiotic therapy

b. Diagnose tuberculosis

c. Differentiate gram-negative and gram-positive bacteria

d. Determine the presence of malignancy

33. A frozen section specimen is not placed in formalin to avoid:

a. Formation of ice crystals

b. Contamination of the specimen

c. Cross-contamination of the laboratory personnel

d. Spillage on the way to the laboratory

34. The procedure in which tissue or fluid is removed for diagnosis is called:

a. An endoscopic surgery procedure

b. A biopsy

c. A Papanicolaou test

d. An aspiration

35. The site used for bone marrow aspiration is usually the:

a. Femur

b. Spinal column

c. Iliac crest

d. Third rib on the right side

36. The procedure done to obtain tissue from internal organs is called:

a. Papanicolaou test

b. Biopsy

c. Acid-fast smear

d. Percutaneous needle biopsy

37. A uterine smear to detect cancer cells in the mucus of the uterus is called a:

a. Biopsy

b. Hormone receptor study

c. Papanicolaou test

d. Percutaneous needle biopsy

38. Human tissue removed for banking may include:

a. Cartilage and hair

b. Bone and nails

c. Skin and hair

d. Cartilage and bone

39. Correctly transporting cultures and specimens to the laboratory is essential for:

a. Time management of personnel

b. Prevention of cross-contamination

c. Continuity of care

d. Life of the tissue

40. Who is responsible for facilitating communication of intraoperative laboratory reports to the surgeon?

a. Nursing assistant

b. Supervisor of the laboratory

c. Scrub nurse

d. Circulating nurse

❖ Answers

1. [c] Potentially infectious

All cultures and specimens should be considered potentially infectious and standard precautions used when collecting and preparing them for examination. Appropriate personal protective equipment should be used as needed. (*page 183*)

2. [b] Material safety data sheets (MSDSs)

Because formalin is designated a hazardous material by federal law, an MSDS is distributed to the purchaser of the chemical. The formalin MSDS should be maintained on file with MSDSs of other hazardous chemicals. (*page 184*)

3. [c] Before the patient is transferred to the operating room bed

To ensure continuity of care, facilitate the procedure, and prevent delays, supplies and equipment needed for cultures and specimens are gathered before the patient is transferred to the procedure room. (*page 184*)

4. [a] Properly label cultures and specimens

Proper labeling of cultures and specimen containers is essential for the prevention of patient injury. (*page 184*)

5. [d] Properly label the specimen

Correct labeling of cultures and specimens ensures that the patient receives the appropriate diagnosis and treatment. (*page 184*)

6. [d] Death

Formalin vapors are toxic. They can cause headaches, coughing, nausea, weakness, pneumonitis, pulmonary edema, and death. In high concentrations, formalin vapors can be fatal. (*page 184*)

7. [b] Ventilate the area

In the event of a formalin spill, one should ventilate the area, remove the sources of ignition, and clean the area according to hospital policy and procedure. (*page 184*)

8. [a] Identify the type of study requested

All laboratory slips have the same purpose: to identify the type of study requested, communicate pertinent patient information to the laboratory, and serve as a reporting document for the attending physician. (*page 185*)

9. [b] Chain of custody

Chain of custody is a mechanism to ensure accountability for cultures and tissue specimens. (*page 185*)

10. [c] Log book

Log books are used to track the specimen from the operative and invasive procedure suite to the laboratory or pathology department. (*page 185*)

11. [d] Identify the pathogen causing the infection

The purpose of the culture is to identify the pathogen causing the infection. The physician uses this information to order appropriate antibiotics and to start a treatment regimen. (*page 186*)

12. [a] Aerobic bacteria

Aerobic bacteria require the presence of oxygen for survival. (*page 186*)

13. [b] Anaerobic bacteria

Anaerobic bacteria grow in the absence of oxygen. (*page 186*)

14. [a] One

If multiple studies are ordered, one specimen is obtained for each container. (*page 186*)

15. [c] *Salmonella*

Gram-negative bacilli include *Escherichia coli, Salmonella, Klebsiella, Pseudomonas, Proteus, Serratia marcescens,* and *Haemophilus influenzae.* (*page 186*)

16. [d] 1 : 10 dilution of household bleach

The tube is decontaminated with a 1 : 10 dilution of household bleach. (*page 187*)

17. [d] 1 : 10 dilution of household bleach

A tuberculocidal hospital-grade disinfectant is a 1 : 10 dilution of household bleach. (*page 187*)

18. [a] Gram stain

A Gram stain is obtained to classify the species of bacteria. Test results guide the physician in initiating appropriate antibiotic therapy. (*page 187*)

19. [b] An aerobic culture tube

Cultures for Gram stains are collected using an aerobic culture tube and are immediately sent to the laboratory for smear and fixation. (*page 187*)

20. [d] Pink

Gram-negative bacteria lose the stain and take the color of the counterstain, which is pink. (*page 187*)

21. [c] Blue

Gram-positive bacteria retain the color of the gentian violet stain, which is blue. (*page 187*)

22. [a] 2.0 mL

Guidelines for minimal amounts of fluids include 1.5–2.0 mL for aerobic culture and smear, 1.0 mL for fungus culture, and 2.0 mL for acid-fast culture and smear. (*page 187*)

23. [b] An acid-fast culture

Acid-fast cultures and smears are done to diagnose tuberculosis. These cultures and smears are sent in the aerobic transport system. (*page 187*)

24. [c] Should not be shaken

All specimens should be handled carefully and as little as possible and should not be shaken. (*page 188*)

25. [d] May rupture the cells

Fluid specimen should not be shaken, since this can rupture the cells. (*page 188*)

26. [a] In a near-natural state

Tissue should remain in a near-natural state, particularly tissue sent for frozen section examination. The work of the pathologist is facilitated if the specimen is received in the same condition as when removed. (*page 188*)

27. [b] Hospital policy

All tissue or other objects removed from the patient are sent to the laboratory as permanent specimens. Exceptions to this guideline are dictated by hospital policy. (*page 188*)

28. [c] Handed off the sterile field as soon as possible

All specimens should be handed off the sterile field as soon as possible to prevent inadvertent discarding of the specimen during cleanup at the end of the procedure. (*page 188*)

29. [a] It prevents decomposition.

Specimens should be completely covered with formalin. Exceptions are bladder and gallstones, which are kept dry to prevent decomposition. (*page 188*)

30. [b] Material that provides contrast

When the size of the specimen makes it difficult to see, the scrub nurse should place it on a piece of material that provides contrast. Telfa dressing pads are suitable and may be submerged in formalin and sent to the laboratory. (*page 188*)

31. [c] Quick preliminary diagnosis

The frozen section examination provides the surgeon with a quick preliminary diagnosis. (*page 188*)

32. [d] Determine the presence of malignancy

Frozen sections are analyzed to determine the presence of malignancy and to identify tissue during the procedure, such as parathyroid tissue and lymph nodes. (*page 188*)

33. [a] Formation of ice crystals

A frozen section specimen should not be placed in fluid such as formalin or saline, because moisture forms ice crystals during the freezing process, which interferes with the examination. (*page 188*)

34. [b] A biopsy

Biopsy refers to a procedure in which tissue or fluid is removed for diagnosis. The physician requests a biopsy to have a definitive diagnosis before further operative intervention or medical treatment is scheduled. (*page 188*)

35. [c] Iliac crest

A skin incision or percutaneous puncture is made; a trocar puncture needle is inserted into the bone, usually the iliac crest or the sternum; and the bone marrow is aspirated. (*page 188*)

36. [d] Percutaneous needle biopsy

Percutaneous needle biopsy is done to obtain tissue from internal organs, such as the liver or the prostate gland. A hollow needle is inserted through the body wall, and the tissue is removed. (*page 188*)

37. [c] Papanicolaou test

The Papanicolaou test, commonly called the Pap smear, is a uterine smear to detect cancer cells in the mucus of the uterus. (*page 189*)

38. [d] Cartilage and bone

The facility should establish guidelines for storing, preserving, and maintaining tissue banks according to the American Association of Tissue Banks. Human tissue removed for banking may include cartilage, bone, and skin. (*page 189*)

39. [c] Continuity of care

Correctly transporting cultures and specimens to the laboratory is essential for continuity of care. The transporter must understand where and to whom the culture or specimen is to be delivered. Assistive personnel responsible for transportation duties should receive specific training in handling cultures and specimens during transportation. (*page 189*)

40. [d] Circulating nurse

The nurse facilitates the communication of laboratory or pathology reports between the physician and the laboratory or the pathology department. (*page 189*)

CHAPTER 13

Handling Tissues With Instruments

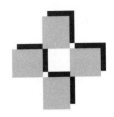

Handling tissues with instruments refers to skills that the registered nurse first assistant (RNFA) uses to provide exposure of the operative site and to clamp, suture, and cut tissue. Because of the fact that tissue is cut, every operation causes injury to the patient. The nurse can minimize this injury by carefully and gently handling tissue and instruments. Correct handling improves the result of any operation, thus minimizing damage and accelerating healing. The questions for this chapter will help the reader assess his or her knowledge about

- Identifying the patient's risk for adverse outcomes related to the handling of tissue with instruments
- Providing exposure during surgery
- Clamping tissue
- Grasping tissue
- Suturing
- Cutting tissue

The reference used for this chapter is Phippen, M. L., & Wells, M. P. (1999). *Patient care during operative and invasive procedures.* Philadelphia: W. B. Saunders, pp. 191–214.

✠ Questions

1. Achieving exposure of the operative site requires:

   a. Aggressive traction

   b. A Penrose drain

   c. Adequate traction

   d. An intestinal bag

2. What can the RNFA use to stabilize and hold anatomical structures?

   a. Laparotomy sponges and towel clamps

   b. Towel clamps and vascular clamps

   c. Self-retaining retractor and laparotomy sponges

   d. 4 × 4 inch radiopaque sponges and laparotomy sponges

3. An example of an instrument designed to dissect tissue and bone is:

   a. Hemostat

   b. Rib approximator

   c. Rongeur

   d. Tenaculum

4. An example of an instrument designed to control bleeding is:

   a. Intestinal clamp

   b. Chisel

   c. Suction tube

   d. Tissue forceps

5. An example of an instrument designed to hold tissue or bone for dissection is:

   a. Artery clamp

   b. Osteotome

   c. Dilator

   d. Tenaculum

6. Handheld retractors were designed to:

   a. Dissect tissue

   b. Maintain hemostasis

   c. Provide the best exposure

   d. Hold tissue for dissection

7. Rose Morgan is a 56-year-old woman admitted to the operating room for an appendectomy. It was discovered that the instruments had not been properly sterilized. The nursing diagnosis would be:

   a. *Potential for Pain related to the surgical procedure*

   b. *Ineffective Coping related to the emergency situation of the surgical procedure*

   c. *Potential for Infection related to handling tissue with instruments during surgery*

   d. *Ineffective Coping related to the hospital experience*

8. Three hours after Max May had a parotidectomy, the incision line is swollen and red. The doctor is concerned that a hematoma is forming. The nursing diagnosis is:

   a. *Risk for Infection related to nutritional deficit*

   b. *Risk for Impaired Tissue Integrity related to poor intraoperative hemostasis*

   c. *Risk for Injury related to excessive retraction*

   d. *Ineffective Coping related to incisional scarring*

9. Postoperative complaints of excessive musculoskeletal pain, neuromuscular impairment, or unexplained fever are suggestive of:

   a. Too small an exposure site

   b. Overly aggressive exposure techniques

   c. Too large an exposure site

   d. Surgical procedure too long

10. Why are 4 × 4 inch radiopaque sponges not used in the abdominal cavity?

   a. Their potential to cause bruising

   b. Their potential to cause slipping of tissue

   c. Their small size

   d. Their absorbability

11. Before packing the abdominal cavity, the scrub nurse must:

   a. Moisten sponges with distilled water

   b. Tack all sponges together with staples

   c. Document the number used for the operating room record

   d. Moisten sponges with warm saline

12. A device used to keep the bowel moist and aid in retaining body heat is called:

   a. Thermal blanket

   b. Moist saline lap sponges

   c. 4 × 4 inch radiopaque sponges

   d. Intestinal bag

13. Stockinet is used in isolating an extremity because it allows the RNFA to:

   a. Hold the extremity without scrubbing

   b. Reposition, hold the extremity, and provide traction

   c. Provide traction and control bleeding

   d. Provide exposure for surgeon and control bleeding

14. What device does the surgeon gently place around tissue to obtain better exposure of the surgical site?

   a. Small pieces of stockinet

   b. Suture stitches

   c. Small retractors

   d. Cotton cord tapes

15. A retractor placed in error can cause:

   a. Excessive tension

   b. Increased visual fluid

   c. Tearing and stretching of blood vessels

   d. Increased fluid pooling

16. If the RNFA uses the wrong type of grasping instrument, the end result could be:

    a. Compression of organs

    b. Underexposure at the surgical site

    c. Increase in fluid pooling

    d. Puncture of delicate tissue

17. Self-retaining retractors with sharp blades are used to hold:

    a. Muscle

    b. Skin

    c. Bone

    d. Nerve

18. Self-retaining retractors with smooth blades are used to hold:

    a. Muscle

    b. Fascia

    c. Subcutaneous tissue

    d. Skin

19. When using retractors, the RNFA must constantly watch for:

    a. Adequate exposure

    b. Tissue blanching

    c. Decrease in fluid pooling

    d. Increased reddened areas

20. An example of a handheld retractor is:

    a. Mueller-Balfour

    b. Lahey goiter

    c. Rochester-Péan

    d. Gomez

21. The act of creating a plane of dissection that opens the connective tissue and provides exposure is:

    a. Traction

    b. Countertraction

    c. Clamping

    d. Dissecting

22. What instrument is the most widely used instrument in surgery?

    a. Lahey goiter

    b. Hemostatic artery forceps

    c. Tissue forceps

    d. Smooth vascular clamps

23. An example of an instrument designed to grasp superficial vessels is:

    a. Osteotome

    b. Sponge forceps

    c. Hemostat

    d. Suction tube

24. What instrument provides hemostasis or partial occlusion until the vessel can be sutured?

    a. Vascular clamp

    b. Hemostatic artery clamp

    c. Adson forceps

    d. Lahey forceps

25. The gentlest of all instruments in a surgical procedure is the:

    a. Fingers

    b. Noncrushing clamps

    c. Vascular clamps

    d. Hemostatic artery forceps

26. What type of forceps would be used on tissue that bleeds easily?

    a. Bayonet forceps

    b. Hemostats

    c. Bulldogs

    d. Smooth-jawed forceps

27. Cushing, Adson, and Singley are all examples of:

    a. Tissue forceps

    b. Dressing forceps

    c. Bayonet forceps

    d. Hemostats

28. Making the incision with one stroke while evenly applying pressure aids in:

    a. Tissue approximation at wound closure

    b. Healing by second intention

    c. Healing by third intention

    d. Formation of granulation tissue

29. Complete hemostasis before wound closure reduces the chance of:

    a. Formation of granulation

    b. Postoperative hematoma formation

    c. Primary union of incised tissue

    d. First-intention healing

30. Foreign bodies (dirt, metal, and glass) left in a wound increase the probability of:

    a. First-intention healing

    b. Second-intention healing

    c. Wound approximation

    d. Wound infection

31. Accurate approximation of tissue without tension or strangulation promotes:

    a. Cavitation

    b. Third-intention healing

    c. Scar formation

    d. First-intention healing

32. First-intention healing occurs by:

    a. Formation of granulation tissue

    b. Primary union of incised tissue

    c. Two surfaces of granulation tissue joining

    d. Grafting of tissue to original surgical site

33. Three days after Marge Vitaz had abdominal surgery, her wound became infected. The wound was left open to aid healing. The process for healing would be:

    a. First intention

    b. Second intention

    c. Third intention

    d. Superficial

34. How long does it take chromic suture to absorb?

    a. 5–70 days

    b. 20–90 days

    c. 40–90 days

    d. 90–200 days

35. Which is an absorbable suture?

    a. Silk

    b. Cotton

    c. Nylon

    d. Polyglactin 910 (Vicryl)

36. When a wound is left open to heal from the bottom up, it is called:

    a. Primary healing

    b. Contraction

    c. Third intention

    d. Approximation

37. The slowest of all healing processes is:

    a. Contraction

    b. First intention

    c. Second intention

    d. Third intention

38. Today, Kristen Hall, the new resident, will be trying to knot nylon suture. What should she know about nylon?

    a. Monofilament requires more knots to prevent slippage.

    b. Monofilament has the potential to cause infection.

    c. It is an absorbable suture.

    d. Multifilament requires more knots to prevent slippage.

39. Sherryle Smith, RNFA, has selected ethibond suture. What are the characteristics of this suture?

    a. Monofilament; potential for harboring infection

    b. Multifilament; knotting is more secure; braiding can harbor bacteria

    c. Monofilament; easy to knot; knot is more secure

    d. Multifilament; requires more knots to prevent slippage

40. Approximation of like tissue (fascia to fascia, skin to skin) and the elimination of all dead space is an example of:

    a. Retention

    b. Primary closure

    c. Secondary closure

    d. Common closure

41. Sutures that are too tight cause:

    a. Blanching and strangulation

    b. Dead space and wide scarring

    c. Infection and granulation

    d. Contamination and coaptation

42. Tissue that heals slowly (skin or tendons) should be closed with:

    a. Absorbable suture

    b. Monofilament suture

    c. Multifilament suture

    d. Nonabsorbable suture

43. Walter Edwards was brought into the operating room for repair of a leg injury sustained in a motor vehicle accident. He had been dragged 20 feet after being hit. The suture of choice for closure would be:

    a. Multifilament

    b. Nonabsorbable

    c. Braided

    d. Monofilament

44. Judy Williams is about to undergo cosmetic surgery. When selecting the suture for this case, the RNFA will select:

    a. Small monofilament

    b. Multifilament

    c. Rapidly absorbed

    d. Staples

45. The technique used to close a tissue layer by passing one strand of suture back and forth between two edges of the wound with a knot at the end is called:

    a. Interrupted

    b. Retention

    c. Horizontal mattress

    d. Running stitch

46. A series of singly placed stitches individually tied and cut is called:

    a. A retention suture

    b. A continuous suture line

    c. An interrupted suture line

    d. An approximated suture line

47. The presence of an infection or gross contamination necessitates:

    a. Secondary closure

    b. Correct approximation

c. Retention sutures

d. Horizontal mattress suture

48. The first stage of a secondary closure is closing the deep tissue. This should be done with:

a. Multifilament suture

b. Monofilament suture

c. Staples

d. Rapidly absorbed suture

49. Part of the wound is left open in a secondary wound closure to allow for:

a. Approximation of wound

b. Granulation of scar tissue

c. Contamination of the wound

d. Periodic installation of antibiotics

50. During secondary wound closure, some surgeons insert skin suture to pull edges together and to:

a. Reduce tension on the incision

b. Prevent contraction

c. Reduce gross contamination

d. Reduce the need for antibiotics

51. In the presence of gross contamination or for obese patients, the surgeon will use:

a. Retention sutures

b. Inverted mattress sutures

c. Skin staples

d. Running stitches

52. When placing retention sutures, the surgeon will use what closure technique?

a. Buried coaptation retention

b. Interrupted mattress

c. Continuous horizontal

d. Continuous over and over

53. To prevent strangulation of the viscera during closure, the RNFA should:

a. Prepare the bolster for safety

b. Prepare the intestinal bag

c. Prepare the solution for irrigation

d. Place his or her finger in the abdominal cavity

54. To prevent a heavy retention suture from cutting into the skin, the surgeon places:

a. Staples

b. Bolsters

c. Skin staples

d. Pursestring suture

55. The RNFA should receive the needle holder from the scrub nurse with the:

a. Needle holder closed to the third ratchet

b. Needle point toward the thumb

c. Needle holder open

d. Needle point away from the thumb

56. The needle should be placed in the needle holder, in the jaws:

a. At the bevel

b. Just before the suture

c. Exactly in the middle

d. Just distal to the flattened area

57. The stitch most commonly used by surgeons to close the abdomen is known as:

a. Smead-Jones

b. Somerville

c. Crile

d. Half stitch

58. What knot is used to maintain proper position of the tissue because it stays in place after the first throw?

 a. Square knot

 b. Granny knot

 c. Slip knot

 d. Surgeon's knot

59. If surgical gut is used, the strand should be cut:

 a. 6 mm from the knot

 b. 4 mm from the knot

 c. 3 mm from the knot

 d. 2 mm from the knot

60. If synthetic suture is used, the strand should be cut:

 a. 1 mm from the knot

 b. 2 mm from the knot

 c. 3 mm from the knot

 d. 4 mm from the knot

61. Why is synthetic suture cut shorter than surgical gut?

 a. To minimize foreign material in wound

 b. Synthetic is stronger

 c. To minimize slippage

 d. To prevent strangulation of the tissue

62. When is the blade of the scalpel changed?

 a. After each use

 b. When the blade becomes dull

 c. Every hour from the start of surgery

 d. Never

63. The scalpel handle is held against the palm with the thumb and fingers

gripping from above in what is known as the:

 a. Power grip

 b. Bard-Parker grip

 c. Precision grip

 d. Pencil grip

64. At what angle should the scalpel be held to allow the sides of the wound to be of equal height and to facilitate proper closure?

 a. 20 degrees

 b. 45 degrees

 c. 70 degrees

 d. 90 degrees

65. What blade has a small curve and cutting edge and is used for small incisions?

 a. No. 10

 b. No. 11

 c. No. 15

 d. No. 20

66. The instrument used for dissecting tissue and severing clamped vessels is the:

 a. Scissors

 b. Scalpel

 c. Hemostat

 d. Lahey

67. Because powered instruments generate heat that can damage surrounding tissue, the RNFA should:

 a. Record the number of minutes the instrument is used

 b. Drip saline onto the blade at intervals to keep the blade cool

 c. Expect the attending physician to be the only one to use powered instruments

d. Keep the suction beside the powered instrument to help keep it cool

68. What knot is used to maintain tension and does not slip after the first throw is in place?

   a. Granny knot

   b. Simple knot

   c. Half-hitch knot

   d. Surgeon's knot

69. When making a deep tie, what can be used to complete the tie?

   a. Bayonet

   b. Needle holder

   c. Sponge forceps

   d. Lahey

70. What blade is used to cut tissue at the bottom of a deep hole?

   a. No. 15 blade

   b. No. 11 blade

   c. Right-angled scalpel blade

   d. Wide-angle blade

71. What is the name of the heated blade that seals small blood vessel as it cuts?

   a. Metzenbaum

   b. Argon beam coagulator

   c. Beaver

   d. Shaw

✚ Answers

1. [c] Adequate traction

   Achieving operative site exposure requires adequate traction. A poorly exposed operative site, because of inadequate retraction, impedes the physician. Overly aggressive traction may cause injury to the patient. (*page 192*)

2. [d] 4 × 4 inch radiopaque sponges and laparotomy sponges

   Laparotomy and 4 × 4 or 4 × 8 inch (10 × 10 or 10 × 20 cm) radiopaque sponges are used to stabilize and hold anatomical structures. (*page 192*)

3. [c] Rongeur

   Examples of instruments designed to incise and dissect tissue and bone include scalpels, scissors, bone cutters, rongeurs, chisels, curets, saws, and osteotomes. (*page 192*)

4. [a] Intestinal clamp

   Examples of instruments designed to control bleeding and maintain hemostasis include hemostats (artery clamps), vascular clamps, and intestinal clamps. These instruments can also be used to grasp or retract tissue. (*page 192*)

5. [d] Tenaculum

   Examples of instruments used to grasp and hold tissue or bone for dissection or retraction or to assist in suturing include tissue forceps, tenacula, rib approximators, sponge forceps, and towel clips. (*page 192*)

6. [c] Provide the best exposure

   Examples of instruments designed to provide the best exposure with minimal trauma to the surrounding tissue include self-retaining and handheld retractors. (*page 192*)

7. [c] *Potential for Infection related to holding tissue with instruments*

   Risk factors associated with *Potential for Infection related to holding tissue with instruments* include immunosuppression, inadequate hemostasis, use of contaminated instruments, and poor approximation of tissues, resulting in the formation of dead space. (*page 193*)

8. [b] *Risk for Impaired Tissue Integrity related to poor intraoperative hemostasis*

The risk factor of poor intraoperative hemostasis is associated with the nursing diagnosis *Risk for Impaired Tissue Integrity.* (*page 193*)

9. [b] Overly aggressive exposure techniques

Excessive musculoskeletal pain, neuromuscular impairment, and unexplained fever after surgery can be associated with overly aggressive exposure technique or an inadvertently punctured organ. (*page 193*)

10. [c] Their small size

Because of the small size of radiopaque sponges, they are not used in the abdominal cavity. Laparotomy sponges provide an excellent means for grasping and holding internal organs such as the large and small intestines. (*page 194*)

11. [d] Moisten sponges with warm saline

When packing the bowel, laparotomy sponges are used. Before packing, the scrub nurse should moisten the sponges with warm normal saline. (*page 194*)

12. [d] Intestinal bag

An intestinal bag keeps the bowel moist, aids in retaining body heat, and protects the bowel from inadvertent abrasion during an extended procedure. When an intestinal bag is in use, the moisture content of the bag and the tissue integrity of the bowel must be monitored. (*page 194*)

13. [b] Reposition, hold the extremity, and provide traction

In isolating an extremity, an impervious stockinet is used to hold, reposition, or provide traction on the extremity during the procedure. (*page 194*)

14. [d] Cotton cord tapes

Tapes, such as cotton cord ties, vessel loops, and Penrose drains, are used to move or hold anatomical structures during the procedure to allow a better view of the operative field. (*page 194*)

15. [c] Tearing and stretching of blood vessels

A misplaced retractor can compress, tear, or stretch blood vessels, nerves, and organs. (*page 195*)

16. [d] Puncture of delicate tissue

The wrong type of grasping instrument can puncture delicate tissue, causing intraoperative and postoperative complications. (*page 195*)

17. [b] Skin

Self-retaining retractors isolate and hold all types of tissue. Blades with sharp or dull teeth hold fasciae, subcutaneous tissue, and skin. (*page 195*)

18. [a] Muscle

Self-retaining retractors with smooth blades are normally used to hold muscle. (*page 195*)

19. [b] Tissue blanching

If signs such as tissue blanching, cessation of pulse, or leaking of fluid appear, exposure methods should be evaluated. (*page 195*)

20. [b] Lahey goiter

Exposure is fine tuned with handheld retractors, such as the Lahey goiter, Green goiter, Senn, US Army, Mayo-Collins, and Volkmann retractors. (*page 195*)

21. [b] Countertraction

When a physician requests exposure, the nurse applies the principles of traction and countertraction. Countertraction creates a plane of dissection that opens the connective tissue and provides exposure. (*page 196*)

22. [b] Hemostatic artery forceps

The most widely used instrument in surgery is the hemostatic artery clamp, which is also called a hemostat. (*page 196*)

23. [c] Hemostat

The hemostat is commonly used to grasp superficial vessels. (*page 196*)

24. [a] Vascular clamp

Vascular clamps provide hemostasis or partial occlusion until the vessel can be sutured. These instruments are available in many shapes and sizes. (*page 196*)

25. [a] Fingers

When possible, the tissue should be lifted with the gentlest of all instruments—the fingers. (*page 197*)

26. [d] Smooth-jawed forceps

Smooth-jawed forceps are used on tissue that would likely bleed or easily perforate, such as bowel and liver tissue. (*page 198*)

27. [b] Dressing forceps

Examples of dressing forceps include Cushing, Adson, and Singley forceps. (*page 198*)

28. [a] Tissue approximation at wound closure

Making the skin incision with one stroke of evenly applied pressure on the scalpel aids in tissue approximation during wound closure. (*page 198*)

29. [b] Postoperative hematoma formation

Complete hemostasis before closing of the wound reduces the chance of hematoma formation. A hematoma or seroma in the incision prevents the direct approximation essential to the union of wound surfaces. (*page 198*)

30. [d] Wound infection

Adequate débridement of all necrotic and devitalized tissue and removal of inflicted foreign bodies promote healing, especially of traumatic wounds. Foreign bodies such as dirt, metal, and glass increase the probability of wound infection. (*page 198*)

31. [d] First-intention healing

Approximation of tissue as nontraumatically as possible without tension or strangulation promotes healing by primary union or first intention. (*page 199*)

32. [b] Primary union of incised tissue

First-intention healing occurs by primary union of the incised tissue. Most patients heal by first intention if tissue damage is minimal during the operation, if aseptic conditions are maintained, if tissue is gently handled, and if dead space is eliminated. (*page 199*)

33. [b] Second intention

Postoperative complications such as wound dehiscence, infection, and excessive scar formation impede first-intention healing and set the stage for second-intention healing. (*page 199*)

34. [b] 20–90 days

Chromic suture is absorbed in 20–90 days. (*page 199*)

35. [d] Polyglactin 910 (Vicryl)

Examples of absorbable suture would include catgut, both plain and chromic, Vicryl, and polydioxanone. (*page 199*)

36. [b] Contraction

When a wound heals by second intention rather than primary union with suture, the wound is left open and allowed to heal from the bottom up. This is called contraction. (*page 199*)

37. [d] Third intention

Third-intention healing is the slowest of all the healing processes. (*page 200*)

38. [a] Monofilament requires more knots to prevent slippage.

Monofilament consists of a single suture strand, so more knots are needed to prevent slippage. (*page 200*)

39. [b] Multifilament; knotting is more secure; braiding can harbor bacteria

Multifilament suture consists of strands of braided suture. It is easier to tie, and the knotting is more secure. A disadvantage, however, is the possible harboring of bacteria in the braided structure of the suture strand. (*page 200*)

40. [b] Primary closure

Primary closure, bringing layers of tissue into approximation (fascia to fascia, muscle to muscle, skin to skin), and the elimination of all dead space allow each layer to heal properly. (*page 200*)

41. [a] Blanching and strangulation

If sutures are too tight, the tissue will blanch then strangulate, causing it to die because of lack of adequate blood supply. Likewise, if sutures slip or become loose, dead space may form and fluid may seep into the wound. (*page 200*)

42. [d] Nonabsorbable suture

Tissue that is slow to heal (skin, fascia, and tendons) should usually be closed with nonabsorbable suture. (*page 200*)

43. [d] Monofilament

Monofilament or absorbable suture is used in potentially contaminated tissues. (*page 200*)

44. [a] Small monofilament

When cosmetic results are important, the smallest inert monofilament suture material should be used, such as nylon or polypropylene. (*page 200*)

45. [d] Running stitch

A continuous suture (running stitch) is used to close a tissue layer by passing one strand of suture back and forth between the two edges of the wound. The physician ties the suture at the end of the suture line. (*page 203*)

46. [c] An interrupted suture line

An interrupted suture line is a series of singly placed stitches. As each suture is placed, it is tied and cut. This technique is used more often than continuous suturing, even though it takes more time, because the integrity of the suture line remains intact if a suture breaks. (*page 203*)

47. [a] Secondary closure

The presence of infection or gross contamination necessitates a secondary closure. This allows access to the contaminated tissue for cleaning and enables the tissue to recover from the infection before final closure. (*page 203*)

48. [b] Monofilament suture

During the first stage of a secondary closure, the deep tissue, such as the peritoneum and fascia, is closed with a monofilament suture material. (*page 203*)

49. [d] Periodic installation of antibiotics

The secondary closure leaves part of the wound open to allow for irrigation of the wound and instillation of antibiotics during dressing changes. (*page 203*)

50. [a] Reduce tension on the incision

Some surgeons insert skin suture during a secondary closure to allow skin edges to pull together and to reduce tension on the incision. (*page 203*)

51. [a] Retention sutures

In the presence of gross contamination, obesity, tissue loss, or excessive tissue damage, such as the type seen with massive trauma, retention sutures are used. (*page 204*)

52. [a] Buried coaptation retention

When placing retention suture, the surgeon selects either through-and-through retention or buried coaptation retention. (*page 204*)

53. [d] Place his or her finger in the abdominal cavity

While tying, the RNFA should place a finger in the abdominal cavity to prevent strangulation of the viscera during closure. Closure of the remainder of the wound continues in a similar manner. (*page 205*)

54. [b] Bolsters

Bolsters are used to prevent the heavy suture material from cutting into the skin. (*page 205*)

55. [b] Needle point toward the thumb

The RNFA receives the needle holder with the needle point toward the thumb. This prevents unnecessary wrist motion. (*page 205*)

56. [d] Just distal to the flattened area

The needle is placed in the jaws just below the point where it flattens out. (*page 206*)

57. [a] Smead-Jones

Many surgeons use the Smead-Jones stitch when closing the abdomen. This stitch approximates peritoneum, muscle, and fascia simultaneously. (*page 206*)

58. [d] Surgeon's knot

Because it usually stays in place after the first throw is made, the surgeon's knot is used to maintain the proper position of the tissue, particularly when one is working in deep tissue. (*page 208*)

59. [a] 6 mm from the knot

If a surgical gut has been used, the strand is cut 6 mm from the knot. (*page 208*)

60. [c] 3 mm from the knot

Synthetic suture is cut 3 mm from the knot. (*page 208*)

61. [a] To minimize foreign material in the wound

Synthetic suture is cut 3 mm from the knot to minimize the amount of foreign material left in the wound. (*page 208*)

62. [b] When the blade becomes dull

The modern scalpel consists of a handle that is designed to receive a variety of disposable blades. The blade of the scalpel should be changed as soon as it becomes dull. (*page 208*)

63. [a] Power grip

The power grip is for large incisions. The scalpel handle is held against the palm, with the thumb and fingers gripping it from above. (*page 208*)

64. [d] 90 degrees

The scalpel should be at a 90-degree angle to the skin. This allows the sides of the wound to be of equal height and facilitates proper closure. (*page 208*)

65. [c] No. 15

A No. 15 blade has a small curve and short cutting surface and is used for small incisions and dissecting fine tissue. The No. 15 blade can also be used with a pencil-like grip. (*page 208*)

66. [a] Scissors

Scissors are used for dissecting tissue, severing clamped blood vessels, and cutting suture. When using scissors, the nurse maintains control by inserting the thumb and fourth finger through the handle rings. The index and third fingers are then used to stabilize the scissors as they cut. (*page 213*)

67. [b] Drip saline onto the blade at intervals to keep the blade cool

Powered tools generate heat and should be used only for short periods. Because heat damages adjunct tissue, cool saline is dripped onto the blade or drill whenever it is being used. (*page 214*)

68. [d] Surgeon's knot

Tension or traction on the tissue is maintained with a surgeon's knot. This knot does not slip after the first throw is in place. (*page 208*)

69. [b] Needle holder

When making a deep tie, a needle holder is used to complete the tie. One loops the suture around the end of the holder, grasps the other end of the suture, and pulls it through the loop. (*page 208*)

70. [c] Right-angled scalpel blade

The right-angled scalpel blade is used to cut tissue at the bottom of a deep hole. (*page 208*)

71. [d] Shaw

The Shaw scalpel is a heated blade that seals small blood vessels as it cuts. This is a slow process and is often used in delicate surgery, such as infertility procedures, in which bleeding must be well controlled. (*page 213*)

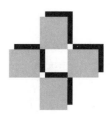

CHAPTER 14

Providing Hemostasis

The term *hemostasis* means prevention of blood loss. Because hemostasis is essential to successful wound management, applying hemostatic techniques is one of the critical tasks done by registered nurse first assistants (RNFAs). The questions for this chapter will help the reader assess his or her knowledge about

- Describing the mechanism of clotting
- Assessing the patient's clotting mechanisms
- Describing the signs of hypovolemic shock
- Identifying the patient's risk for adverse outcomes related to the provision of hemostasis
- Applying mechanical methods to control bleeding
- Applying thermal methods to control bleeding
- Applying chemical methods to control bleeding

The reference used for this chapter is Phippen, M. L., & Wells, M. P. (1999). *Patient care during operative and invasive procedures.* Philadelphia: W. B. Saunders, pp. 215–226.

Questions

1. The prevention of blood loss is:
    a. Clotting
    b. Hypotension
    c. Hemostasis
    d. Shock

2. The person responsible for determining the appropriate hemostatic technique is the:
    a. Circulating nurse
    b. Scrub nurse
    c. RNFA
    d. Surgeon

3. When a blood vessel is cut, it:
    a. Contracts
    b. Constricts
    c. Spasms
    d. Crushes

4. Direct trauma to the muscle wall causes it to:
    a. Contract
    b. Constrict
    c. Spasm
    d. Crush

5. After damage to the blood vessel is incurred, plugging of the disrupted vessel begins with:
    a. Red blood cells (RBCs)
    b. Platelets
    c. White blood cells (WBCs)
    d. Fibrin

6. Which of the following is *not* a step in blood clot formation?
    a. Vitamin K is depleted.
    b. Prothrombin activators form in response to vessel trauma.
    c. Aided by activators, prothrombin is converted to thrombin.

d. Thrombin converts fibrinogen to fibrin.

7. The studies ordered when the patient's history suggests bleeding or clotting difficulties are:

   a. WBC and RBC count

   b. Prothrombin time and RBC count

   c. Prothrombin time and WBC count

   d. Prothrombin time and partial thromboplastin time

8. Thrombocytopenia develops with:

   a. Increased platelet production

   b. Decreased platelet production

   c. Increased RBCs

   d. Increased WBCs

9. An example of an antiplatelet drug is:

   a. Aspirin

   b. Cold medicine

   c. Antiepileptic drugs

   d. Vitamins

10. Parenteral administration of vitamin K can improve clotting times within:

    a. 8–12 hours

    b. 3–4 hours

    c. 6–10 hours

    d. 1–2 hours

11. Risk factors for disseminated intravascular coagulation include all of the following except:

    a. Hypotension

    b. Widespread metastatic disease

    c. Massive trauma or burns

d. Gram-negative or gram-positive sepsis

12. The amount of blood loss necessary to put the patient at risk for mild hypovolemic shock is:

    a. 10%

    b. 20%

    c. 20%–40%

    d. More than 40%

13. What is the first sign of hypovolemia?

    a. Skin pallor

    b. Tachycardia

    c. Increased urine output

    d. Hypertension

14. The amount of blood loss that would put the patient at risk for moderate shock is:

    a. 10–20%

    b. 20–40%

    c. 30–40%

    d. Over 50%

15. Signs of severe shock include all of the following except:

    a. Hypotension

    b. Tachycardia

    c. Oliguria

    d. Increased urine output

16. The hemostatic mechanism that usually works, regardless of the rate of blood flow and whether it is from a denuded surface or a pulsating artery, is:

    a. Mechanical

    b. Chemical

    c. Thermal

    d. Shaw scalpel

17. Another name for the direct or indirect exertion of force on a surface to stop bleeding is:

    a. Pressure

    b. Clips

    c. Suture

    d. All of the above

18. Mr. Wheeler underwent a radical prostatectomy. He lost 3000 mL of blood during surgery, which lasted 5 hours. The nursing diagnosis that would be most appropriate is:

    a. *Risk for Fluid Volume Deficit related to intraoperative blood loss*

    b. *Risk for Injury related to mechanical methods of hemostasis used intraoperatively*

    c. *Risk for Infection related to length of surgery*

    d. *Risk for Injury related to size of bed in the operating room*

19. Risk factors associated with the use of hemostatic clips to achieve intraoperative hemostasis include:

    a. Poor operative exposure and excessive body hair

    b. Poor tissue mass and scar tissue

    c. Poor operative exposure and adhesions

    d. Adhesions, scar tissue, and excessive body hair

20. Risk factors for infection related to the use of electrosurgery include:

    a. Existing infection, contaminated wound, and immunosuppression (secondary to blood transfusions)

    b. Contaminated wound, immunosuppression (secondary to blood transfusions), and use of inflammable drapes

    c. Existing infection, immunosuppression (secondary to blood transfusions), and use of inflammable drapes

    d. Immunosuppression (secondary to blood transfusions), use of reflective instruments, and poor exposure of the operative site

21. When preparing to use clip appliers, the scrub nurse should have:

    a. Tissue forceps, suction, clips, clip appliers

    b. Tissue forceps, clip appliers, clips

    c. Lap sponges, suction, clip appliers, clips

    d. Clip appliers, clips

22. Two types of thermal methods to control bleeding are:

    a. Electrical current and suture ligature

    b. Laser and hemoclips

    c. Suture ligature and hemoclips

    d. Laser and electrical current

23. The vessels best controlled with thermal hemostasis are:

    a. Large vessels

    b. Medium vessels

    c. Microvessels

    d. Small vessels

24. The blend mode on the electrosurgical unit (ESU) will allow the RNFA to:

    a. Cut through tissue

    b. Cut through tissue while stopping bleeding

    c. Stop bleeding and suction

    d. Suction and cut at the same time

25. The coagulation mode on an ESU achieves hemostasis by:

    a. Exposing tissue

    b. Sealing blood vessels with heat

    c. Sealing blood vessels with cold

    d. A combination of exposing the vessels and sealing the vessels with cold

26. The equipment needed for electrosurgery includes:

    a. Dry laparotomy sponges, ESU, active electrode

    b. Wet laparotomy sponges, scissors, ESU

    c. Dry laparotomy sponges, ESU

    d. Wet laparotomy sponges, forceps, ESU, active electrode

27. Hemostasis with electrosurgery is not as reliable as ties and suture ligatures. Therefore, ESU should be used on:

    a. Microsize vessels

    b. Small vessels

    c. Large vessels

    d. Medium vessels

28. The common sites electrosurgery burns are found on patients include:

    a. Under electrocardiogram (ECG) leads, where drapes touch patient, and temperature probe entry site

    b. Site of dispersive pad, under ECG leads, and where drapes touch patient

    c. Site of patient return electrode, under ECG leads, and temperature probe entry site

    d. Temperature probe site only

29. Carbon dioxide, argon, and neodymium: yttrium-aluminum-garnet (Nd:YAG) are all types of:

    a. ESUs

    b. Forceps

    c. Trocars

    d. Lasers

30. The responsibilities of the circulator during laser surgery include:

    a. Placing warning signs on doors, using inflammable drapes, and using dry sponges

    b. Giving protective glasses to all people in the room and using inflammable agents to prepare the operative site

    c. Preparing reflective instruments, giving protective glasses to everyone in the room, and placing warning signs on doors

    d. Applying saline moistened pads to the patient's eyes, placing warning signs on doors, and giving protective glasses to everyone in the room

31. Instruments used in laser surgery should be:

    a. Bright and reflective

    b. Dull and nonreflective

    c. Dull and reflective

    d. Bright and nonreflective

32. The heat cutting blade of the Shaw scalpel achieves hemostasis by:

    a. Clipping vessels

    b. Cryoprecipitation

    c. Heat sealing

    d. All of the above

33. Documentation on the intraoperative record when the plasma scalpel is in use includes:

    a. Placement of dispersive pad and thermal burns (if present)

    b. Placement of dispersive pad, thermal burns (if present), and safety precautions

c. Thermal burns (if present) and unit number

d. All of the above

34. A chemical agent would be the hemostatic agent of choice when the wound class is:

a. Contaminated

b. Clean

c. Infected

d. Perforated

35. Avitene is a microfibrillar collagen. Its usefulness as a hemostatic agent is that:

a. Platelets are attracted to the bleeding surface and adhere to it

b. It can absorb four to six times its weight

c. It can cause pressure of the bleeding areas

d. All of the above

36. Microfibrillar collagen hemostatic agents may cause wound infection or abscesses because:

a. They are a foreign substance

b. The patient has an allergy to dairy products

c. The RNFA fails to remove the excess collagen from the skin edges

d. None of the above

37. When microfibrillar collagen is used and pressure is applied, hemostasis usually occurs in:

a. 1 minute

b. 5 minutes

c. 30 seconds

d. 5–10 seconds

38. Ellen is having abdominal surgery. The surgeon decides to use a microfibrillar collagen hemostatic agent. The circulator will:

a. Discontinue use of blood-scavenging equipment

b. Initiate use of blood-scavenging equipment

c. Contact the blood bank about the use of microfibrillar collagen

d. Send for a technician to draw arterial blood gases

39. Pliable sponge of purified gelatin that can hold several times its weight is called:

a. Plasma spatula

b. Gelfoam

c. Atavan

d. Electrosurgery

40. What equipment and supplies are needed when using gelfoam?

a. Straight Mayo scissors, dry tissue forceps, suction

b. Dry tissue forceps free from blood, suction, Metzenbaum scissors

c. Suction, wet laparotomy sponges

d. Wet laparotomy sponges, Metzenbaum scissors, suction

41. Gelatin sponges would not be used:

a. On abdominal surgery cases or amputations

b. On cardiovascular and ophthalmological cases

c. On neurosurgery cases, for tendon repair, or in the presence of infection

d. On orthopedic or plastic surgery cases

42. Application of suction to the laparotomy sponge while a gelatin sponge is held in place is done to:

a. Provide a dry area for hemostasis

b. Provide pressure needed for hemostasis

c. Prevent recurrent bleeding

d. Draw blood into the gelatin and hasten clotting

43. The type of hemostatic agent that is a purified and lyophilized (freeze-dried) bovine collagen is:

a. Microfibrillar collagen

b. Collagen sponge

c. Gelatin sponge

d. All of the above

44. Collagen sponges absorb fluid and may expand, exerting pressure on adjacent structures. They should not be used on:

a. Cardiovascular, neurosurgical, and general cases

b. Plastic, general, and cardiovascular cases

c. Neurological, urological, and ophthalmological cases

d. Orthopedic and urological cases

45. The most serious side effects of collagen sponges are:

a. Allergies, excessive bleeding, and hematomas

b. Adhesions, bleeding, and decreased clotting

c. Decreased clotting, allergies, and decreased wound healing

d. Adhesions, allergies, and foreign body reaction

46. The equipment needed for collagen sponge use includes:

a. Straight Mayo scissors, dry forceps, laparotomy sponges, and suction

b. Dry forceps and wet laparotomy sponges

c. Suction, wet laparotomy sponges, and dry forceps

d. Metzenbaum scissors and wet laparotomy sponges

47. After application of a collagen sponge, how much later will hemostasis occur?

a. 2–5 minutes

b. 1 minute

c. 5–8 minutes

d. 15–30 seconds

48. Another name for oxidized cellulose (a white, knitted fabric) is:

a. Gelfoam

b. Surgicel

c. Hemopad

d. All of the above

49. Hemostatic agents that should not be put into an autoclave include:

a. Oxidized cellulose and collagen sponges, and staples

b. Gelatin and collagen sponges, and plasma scalpel handle

c. Microfibrillar collagen and oxidized cellulose, and laser handpiece

d. Oxidized cellulose, collagen sponges, and gelatin sponges

50. Oxidized cellulose should not be used on fractured bones because:

a. It prevents healing

b. It interferes with callus formation

c. It increases surgery time

d. None of the above

51. Oxidized cellulose should be used only:

a. In the presence of whole blood

b. When there is oozing of body fluids

c. As packing material

d. All of the above

52. What equipment is needed when using oxidized cellulose?

    a. ESU unit and a unit of blood in the room

    b. Straight Mayo scissors, suction, and an ESU unit

    c. Straight Mayo scissors, suction, dry laparotomy sponge, and dry forceps

    d. Curved Mayo scissors, suction, and damp laparotomy sponge

53. Before using oxidized cellulose, collagen or gelatin sponges the surgeon should:

    a. Consider mechanical and thermal hemostatic agents

    b. Provide additional exposure

    c. Check the resterilization date for expiration

    d. Wet the cellulose for better absorption

54. The postoperative nurse should be informed when what hemostatic agent is used for packing or is applied to wound surfaces?

    a. Oxidized cellulose

    b. Gelatin sponges

    c. Collagen sponges

    d. Microfibrillar collagen

■ Answers

1. [c] Hemostasis

The term *hemostasis* means prevention of blood loss. Providing hemostasis is an ongoing process throughout the operative or invasive procedure. (*page 215*)

2. [d] Surgeon

Usually, the surgeon determines the appropriate hemostatic technique. The RNFA performs or assists in performing the technique. (*page 215*)

3. [a] Contracts

Depending on the type of trauma, a blood vessel either contracts or constricts when damaged. If cut, a blood vessel contracts. (*page 215*)

4. [b] Constrict

Direct trauma to the muscle in the vessel wall causes it to constrict for several centimeters, resulting in vascular spasm. The greater the trauma, the greater the degree of vasospasm. (*page 215*)

5. [b] Platelets

After damage is incurred, plugging of the disrupted vessel with platelets begins. Platelets are normally oval or round disks. When platelets contract the collagen fibers of a damaged vessel wall, they swell and assume irregular shapes with protuberances. (*page 215*)

6. [a] Vitamin K is depleted.

The steps to form a blood clot are as follows: prothrombin activators form in response to vessel trauma; aided by the activators, prothrombin is converted to thrombin; and thrombin converts the fibrinogen to fibrin. (*page 215*)

7. [d] Prothrombin time and partial thromboplastin time

Prothrombin time and partial thromboplastin time are ordered if a patient has a history of bleeding or clotting difficulties. Prothrombin time measures the extrinsic clotting mechanism. Partial thromboplastin time measures the activity of the intrinsic clotting mechanism. (*page 215*)

8. [b] Decreased platelet production

Thrombocytopenia develops with decreased platelet production, as in bone marrow aplasia, infiltration, suppression (by drugs or radiation), or vitamin B_{12} deficiency. (*page 216*)

9. [a] Aspirin

Qualitative platelet defects should be suspected if the patient takes antiplatelet drugs.

An antiplatelet drug such as aspirin prolongs bleeding time. This effect can last up to 3–5 days. (*page 216*)

10. [a] 8–12 hours

Parenteral administration of vitamin K improves clotting time within 8–12 hours. In the presence of liver disease, however, the degree to which it helps the patient depends on the extent of parenchymal cell damage. (*page 216*)

11. [a] Hypotension

Risk factors associated with disseminated intravascular coagulation include widespread metastatic disease, massive trauma or burns, gram-negative or gram-positive sepsis, and some viral and malarial infections. (*page 216*)

12. [b] 20%

A patient experiencing mild hypovolemic shock has lost up to 20% of blood volume. (*page 216*)

13. [a] Skin pallor

Signs of hypovolemia include poor tissue profusion, especially in the feet, which may be pale, cool, and clammy. If the patient is in the supine position, the blood pressure and pulse remain normal. If sitting, the pulse increases and the blood pressure falls. (*page 217*)

14. [b] 20%–40%

In moderate shock, the patient has lost 20%–40% of circulating blood volume. He or she may have pale skin and a low urine output. (*page 216*)

15. [d] Increased urine output

Hypotension, oliguria, and tachycardia indicate that the patient has lost 40% or more of blood volume and is experiencing severe shock. (*page 216*)

16. [a] Mechanical

Pressure, hemostatic clips, clamps, and sutures are mechanical ways to control bleed-ing. Regardless of the rate of blood flow and whether it is from a denuded surface or a pulsatile artery, mechanical methods usually work. (*page 217*)

17. [a] Pressure

Pressure is the direct or indirect exertion of force on a surface to stop bleeding. Direct pressure is applied with one or more fingers at the site of bleeding. Indirect pressure uses the fingers or palm to compress the area adjacent to the site of active bleeding. (*page 217*)

18. [a] *Risk for Fluid Volume Deficit related to intraoperative blood loss*

Risk factors for fluid volume deficit include bleeding during and after the procedure related to alteration in clotting mechanisms, bleeding during the procedure, hematoma development, and excessive wound drainage. (*page 218*)

19. [c] Poor operative exposure and adhesions

Risk factors associated with hemostatic clips include adhesions, obesity, poor operative exposure, use of packs to stop bleeding, and application of inappropriate-sized clips. (*page 218*)

20. [a] Existing infection, contaminated wound, and immunosuppression (secondary to blood transfusions)

Risk factors associated with the use of ESU include existing infection, contaminated wound, immunosuppression associated with blood transfusion, and hematoma formation due to inadequate cauterization of blood vessels. (*page 219*)

21. [b] Tissue forceps, clip appliers, clips

The equipment and supplies needed for clip application are tissue forceps, clip appliers, and clips. (*page 221*)

22. [d] Laser and electrical current

Electrical current and laser are two methods to thermally control bleeding. (*page 221*)

23. [d] Small vessels

Thermal methods of hemostasis effectively control bleeding from small blood vessels and denuded surfaces. These methods are not reliable for controlling large venous or large pulsating arterial bleeding. (*page 221*)

24. [b] Cut through tissue while stopping bleeding

The blend mode on an ESU machine is used to cut tissue while stopping bleeding. The blended mode uses the cut waveform to achieve the clinical effect. (*page 222*)

25. [b] Sealing blood vessels with heat

When the physician uses the coagulation mode (an intermittent waveform), the generator modifies the waveform to a duty cycle of 6%, which produces less heat. Instead of cutting tissue, this produces a coagulum. (*page 222*)

26. [a] Dry laparotomy sponges, ESU, active electrode

Equipment and supplies needed for electrosurgery include dry laparotomy sponges, appropriate tissue forceps, the electrosurgical generator, a nonconductive holster device to contain and confine the active electrode when not in use, a coated electrode tip, a scratch pad when uncoated electrodes are used, and a patient return electrode for the monopolar procedure. (*page 222*)

27. [b] Small vessels

Hemostasis with electrosurgery is not as reliable as ties or suture ligatures; therefore, it should be used only on small vessels. Hemostasis of large vessels must be accomplished with ties, clips, or suture ligatures. (*page 222*)

28. [c] Site of patient return electrode, under ECG leads, and temperature probe entry site

Ground reference generators are capable of causing a patient burn at alternate pathway sites and at the patient return electrode site. (*page 222*)

29. [d] Lasers

Laser is an acronym for *light amplification by stimulated emission of radiation.* Carbon dioxide, argon, and Nd:YAG are all used to create the laser beam. Each substance produces a different light with its own specific wavelength. (*page 223*)

30. [d] Applying saline moistened pads to the patient's eyes, placing warning signs on doors, and giving protective glasses to everyone in the room

The equipment and supplies needed for laser procedures include damp laparotomy sponges; dull, nonreflective instruments; and appropriate eye protection devices that stop beam transmission. (*page 223*)

31. [b] Dull and nonreflective

Instruments used in laser surgery should be dull and nonreflective. (*page 223*)

32. [c] Heat sealing

The heated cutting blade of the plasma scalpel achieves hemostasis by heat sealing the blood vessels as they are cut. (*page 213*)

33. [c] Thermal burns (if present) and unit number

Plasma scalpel use is documented by including the unit number in the nurse's notes. If thermal burns occur, this must be recorded. (*page 224*)

34. [b] Clean

The nurse should consider wound classification before using a chemical agent because the use of most agents is ill-advised or contraindicated in contaminated wounds. (*page 224*)

35. [a] Platelets are attracted to a bleeding surface and adhere to it.

When a microfibrillar collagen hemostat comes into contact with a bleeding surface, platelets are attracted to it and adhere to the fibrils. The platelets then aggregate, beginning the clotting phenomenon. (*page 224*)

36. [a] They are a foreign substance

Because they are a foreign substance, a microfibrillar collagen hemostat may potentiate wound infections and formation of abscesses. (*page 224*)

37. [a] 1 minute

Hemostasis usually occurs within 1 minute of placement of microfibrillar collagen. The time can vary, depending on the force and severity of the bleeding. Three to 5 minutes may be required for brisk bleeding, such as splenic lacerations or arterial suture lines. (*page 225*)

38. [a] Discontinue use of blood-scavenging equipment

The circulating nurse is notified to discontinue the use of bleed-scavenging equipment once a microfibrillar collagen hemostat is used. An unused microfibrillar collagen hemostat is discarded, not resterilized. (*page 225*)

39. [b] Gelfoam

Gelfoam sponge is a pliable sponge of purified gelatin that can hold several times its weight in blood. (*page 225*)

40. [a] Straight Mayo scissors, dry tissue forceps, suction

Equipment and supplies needed when using gelfoam include straight Mayo scissors, dry tissue forceps, dry laparotomy sponge, suction, and gelatin sponge. (*page 225*)

41. [c] On neurosurgery cases, for tendon repair, or in the presence of infection

Gelatin sponges would not be used on neurosurgery cases, for tendon repair, or in the presence of infection. Before using gelatin sponges, one should evaluate the effectiveness of hemostasis by mechanical and thermal methods. (*page 225*)

42. [d] Draws blood into the gelatin and hastens clotting

An alternative method of using wet or dry gelatin sponge is to apply suction to the laparotomy sponge while holding the gelatin in place. This technique draws blood into the gelatin and seems to hasten clotting. (*page 225*)

43. [b] Collagen sponge

The collagen sponge is a purified and lyophilized bovine dermal collagen. It is prepared as a lightly cross-linked spongelike pad. (*page 225*)

44. [c] Neurological, urological, and ophthalmological cases

Because collagen sponges absorb fluid and may expand, exerting pressure on adjacent structures, they are not recommended for use in neurological, urological, or ophthalmological surgical procedures. (*page 225*)

45. [d] Adhesions, allergies, and foreign body reaction

The most serious side effects of collagen sponges use are formation of adhesions, allergies, and foreign body reactions. (*page 225*)

46. [a] Straight Mayo scissors, dry forceps, laparotomy sponges, and suction

The equipment and supplies needed when using collagen sponges include straight Mayo scissors, dry forceps, laparotomy sponges, and suction. Heating inactivates collagen sponges. (*page 225*)

47. [a] 2–5 minutes

Hemostasis will occur 2–5 minutes after application of collagen sponges. Excessive collagen is removed and collagen is kept away from skin edges when the wound is closed. Unused gelatin sponges should be discarded, not resterilized. (*page 226*)

48. [b] Surgicel

Surgicel, another name for oxidized cellulose, is an absorbable, white, knitted fabric, which has a faint caramel odor. It can be sutured or cut without fraying. (*page 226*)

49. [d] Oxidized cellulose, collagen sponges, and gelatin sponges

Oxidized cellulose, collagen sponges, gelatin sponges, and microfibrillar collagen should not be placed in an autoclave. (*page 226*)

50. [b] It interferes with callus formation

Oxidized cellulose interferes with the formation of calluses. Therefore, it should not be used on bone fractures. Additionally, it absorbs fluid and may expand, exerting pressure on adjacent structures. (*page 226*)

51. [a] In the presence of whole blood

Oxidized cellulose should be used only in the presence of whole blood. Oozing of other body fluids, such as serum, does not react with oxidized cellulose to produce satisfactory hemostasis. (*page 226*)

52. [c] Straight Mayo scissors, suction, dry laparotomy sponges, and dry forceps

The equipment and supplies needed when using oxidized cellulose include straight Mayo scissors, dry tissue forceps (free from blood), dry laparotomy sponges, and suction. (*page 226*)

53. [a] Consider mechanical and thermal hemostatic agents

Before oxidized cellulose, collagen sponges, or gelatin sponges are used, thermal and mechanical hemostatic agents, such as hemoclips and stick ties, should be considered. (*page 226*)

54. [a] Oxidized cellulose

The nurse should be notified when oxidized cellulose is used for packing the surgical incision or is applied to wound surfaces. The nurse should observe for burning and stinging after the removal of a nasal polyp, hemorrhoidectomy, and application to wound surfaces such as donor sites, venous stasis ulcerations, and dermabrasion. If it is causing the patient difficulty, removal is recommended. (*page 226*)

CHAPTER 15

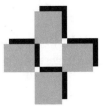

Facilitating Care After the Operative or Invasive Procedure

Facilitating care after the operative or invasive procedure refers to the activities done by the registered nurse during the postprocedure period to make the patient physically and psychologically ready to begin convalescence and rehabilitation. The following questions help the reader assess his or her knowledge about

- Identifying the critical variables that affect the patient's convalescence
- Describing the stages of wound healing
- Recognizing postprocedure wound complications
- Recognizing systemic postprocedure complications
- Assessing the patient's physiological and psychological comfort levels
- Ensuring the proper functioning of devices employed to assist recovery

The reference used for this chapter is Phippen, M. L., & Wells, M. P. (1999). *Patient care during operative and invasive procedures.* Philadelphia: W. B. Saunders, pp. 229–247.

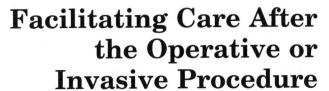

Questions

1. When does the postoperative phase of care begin?

   a. On admission to the postanesthesia care unit (PACU)

   b. When the dressing is applied

   c. On entering the operating room

   d. On leaving the hospital

2. When does postoperative care end?

   a. When the patient leaves the operating room

   b. With the resolution of postoperative sequellae

   c. When the patient leaves the hospital

   d. When the patient is discharged from the physician's care

3. What should be in the report to the PACU nurse?

   a. Pulmonary status, drug allergies, food preferences

   b. Drug allergies, type of surgery, pulmonary status

   c. Type of surgery, names of dependent children

   d. Age of dependent children, food preferences

4. How long does inflammation last in a clean surgical wound?

   a. Several days

   b. 3–5 days

   c. 12 hours

   d. There never should be signs of inflammation

5. How long does it take for wound epithelialization to take place?

   a. 24 hours

   b. 48 hours

   c. 5 days

   d. 1 week

6. How long after the invasive procedure does the cellular phase of wound healing begin?

   a. 1 week

   b. 12 hours

   c. 2–3 days

   d. 6 hours

7. With what phase of wound healing does protein deficiency interfere?

   a. None

   b. Inflammation

   c. Maturation

   d. All phases

8. What vitamin is essential for the synthesis of clotting factor?

   a. Vitamin C

   b. Vitamin K

   c. Vitamin E

   d. Vitamin B_{12}

9. What drugs delay wound healing?

   a. Chemotherapeutic agents, anticoagulants

   b. Morphine, meperidine (Demerol)

   c. Epilepsy drugs

   d. Antibiotics, antiarrhythmic agents

10. On what postoperative days will signs of a urinary tract infection most likely appear?

    a. Days 1–2

    b. Days 8–10

    c. Days 7–9

    d. Days 3–5

11. What are the signs of a wound infection?

    a. Scaled skin edges, no fever, no appetite

    b. No appetite, increased sodium levels

    c. Chills and fever, skin warm to the touch

    d. No appetite, chills and fever

12. If the correct antibiotic is administered, how much later would the condition of the wound improve?

    a. 5 days

    b. 24 hours

    c. 7 days

    d. 12 hours

13. What forms when the inflammatory process becomes suppurative, is confined within a single anatomical space, and is surrounded by granulation tissue?

    a. Gas gangrene

    b. Wound dehiscence

    c. Hematoma

    d. Abscess

14. The abscess area is usually:

    a. Tender

    b. Asymptomatic

    c. Hypersensitive

    d. Very painful

15. What is the treatment of choice for an abscess?

    a. Antibiotic therapy

    b. Warm saline soaks

    c. Drainage of the abscess

    d. Leaving it alone

16. Presence of pus in the wound is a risk factor associated with:

    a. Impaired tissue integrity related to abscess formation

    b. Infection related to seroma formation

c. Potential infection

d. Impaired skin integrity: nonhealing wound

17. Mrs. Thomas' abdominal incision has just undergone culture for *Clostridium perfringens*. The most appropriate nurse diagnosis would be:

   a. *Risk for Impaired Skin Integrity: nonhealing wound*

   b. *Risk for Impaired Tissue Integrity related to abscess formation*

   c. *Risk for Impaired Tissue Integrity related to the formation of gas gangrene*

   d. *Risk for Wound Infection*

18. Mr. Bates is a postoperative patient who had a right inguinal hernia repair. He has insulin-dependent diabetes and is 50 lb overweight. The most appropriate nursing diagnosis would be:

   a. *Risk for Postoperative Hyperthermia*

   b. *Risk for Impaired Skin Integrity related to the formation of gas gangrene*

   c. *Risk for Potential for Infection related to wound dehiscence or evisceration*

   d. *Risk for Impaired Skin Integrity: nonhealing wound*

19. Mrs. Rice takes 0.125 mg digoxin every day for her cardiac problems. She forgot to list digoxin on her medication list when she was admitted to the hospital. Since she has been in the hospital recuperating from her right total hip replacement, she has not taken this medication. The most appropriate nursing diagnosis would be:

   a. *Risk for Alterations in Postoperative Cardiac Rate*

   b. *Risk for Ineffective Airway Clearance*

   c. *Risk for Ineffective Breathing Patterns*

   d. *Risk for Acute Pulmonary Embolus*

20. One of the reasons a patient would have an ineffective breathing pattern during the postprocedure period would be:

   a. The patient's temperature is 36°C (96.8°F)

   b. The physician has ordered complete bed rest for the patient

   c. The patient has a urinary tract infection

   d. The patient smokes two packs of cigarettes a day

21. Urinary retention and dehydration are risk factors associated with:

   a. Postoperative urinary tract infection

   b. Ineffective breathing patterns

   c. Acute pulmonary embolus

   d. Hypoventilation

22. Narcotics given for pain control can be a risk factor for:

   a. Acute pulmonary embolus

   b. Ineffective airway clearance

   c. Altered postprocedure bowel function

   d. Ineffective breathing pattern

23. What type of patient is at an especially high risk for all postoperative pulmonary complications?

   a. Child

   b. Elderly

   c. Nonsmoker

   d. Smoker

24. What are the risk factors associated with seromas?

   a. Malnourished patient, skin flaps

   b. Geriatric patient, small incision

   c. Malnourished patient, small incision

   d. Obese patient, surgical wound with undermined skin flaps

25. What supplies are necessary to aspirate a seroma?

    a. 20–35-mL syringe, 16-gauge needle, skin preparation solution

    b. 3-mL syringe, 27-gauge needle, skin preparation solution

    c. Tuberculosis syringe, ½-inch needle, skin preparation solution

    d. 5-mL syringe, 25-gauge needle, skin preparation solution

26. How many processes are there for gas gangrene?

    a. One

    b. Two

    c. Three

    d. Four

27. How many types of gas gangrene are there?

    a. One

    b. Two

    c. Three

    d. Four

28. Wound dehiscence would most likely be seen on the:

    a. 1st postoperative day

    b. 5th postoperative day

    c. 7th postoperative day

    d. 10th postoperative day

29. The treatment for wound dehiscence or evisceration is:

    a. Antibiotics

    b. Drainage

    c. Surgical closure

    d. Pressure dressing

30. Mr. Brown's abdominal incision has eviscerated. What position will be most appropriate for him?

    a. Prone

    b. Supine

    c. Left lateral

    d. High Fowler's

31. What type of fever is considered normal postoperatively?

    a. Normal

    b. Spiking high

    c. Hypothermic

    d. Transient low-grade

32. Spiking of temperature during the first 2 days postoperatively is usually pulmonary in nature. What would be the primary treatment?

    a. Bed rest

    b. Antibiotics

    c. Ambulation

    d. All of the above

33. What is the major cause of ineffective cough?

    a. Fever

    b. Pain and splinting

    c. Restlessness

    d. Age of the patient

34. Postoperative pulmonary complications usually appear:

    a. 12 hours after the procedure

    b. The first postoperative day

    c. 2 days after the procedure

    d. 4 days after the procedure

35. The cause of segmental atelectasis is:

    a. Bed rest

    b. Inadequate pain medication

c. Early ambulation

d. History of smoking

36. If pneumonia develops as the result of persistent segmental atelectasis or ineffective cough, what would be the added treatment?

a. Antibiotics

b. Mucolytic agents

c. Aspirin

d. Narcotics

37. What is the most common cause of pleural effusion?

a. Pain

b. Pneumonia

c. Type of operation

d. Age of the patient

38. Congestive heart failure postoperatively can be caused by:

a. Early ambulation

b. Intraoperative transfusions

c. Fluid overload

d. Urinary tract infection

39. The inability of the heart to pump enough blood to meet the body's metabolic needs is called:

a. Tachycardia

b. Pneumonia

c. Pulmonary embolus

d. Congestive heart failure

40. What is the first treatment for segmental atelectasis?

a. Bed rest

b. Increased activity

c. Antibiotic therapy

d. Bronchoscopy

41. The treatment for a patient with overhydration is:

a. Diuretics and inotropic drugs

b. Narcotics and diuretics

c. Inotropic drugs and narcotics

d. Diuretics and mucolytic drugs

42. What is the treatment for subdiaphragmatic abscess?

a. Antibiotic therapy

b. Surgical and percutaneous drainage

c. Increased ambulation and aspiration

d. Increased pain medication

43. What causes thrombophlebitis?

a. Inactivity with venous stasis in the lower extremities, poor cough reflex

b. Complication of intravenous catheters, nothing-by-mouth (NPO) status

c. Prolonged venous cannulation, NPO status

d. Prolonged venous cannulation, inactivity with venous stasis in the lower extremities

44. Where does the most serious form of thrombophlebitis occur?

a. Deep veins of upper extremities

b. Superficial veins of upper extremities

c. Deep veins of legs

d. Superficial veins of legs

45. Thrombophlebitis is prevented by maintaining high venous flow. How is this accomplished?

a. Application of elastic stockings, bed rest

b. Elevation of legs, decreased ambulation

c. Muscular exercise, placing legs in a dependent position

d. Application of elastic stockings, elevation of the legs

46. What drug could be ordered for a patient with thrombophlebitis?

a. Heparin

b. Penicillin

c. Meperidine

d. Insulin

47. What are the first signs of returning bowel function?

a. Decreased bowel sounds, increased pain

b. Excessive pain, increased flatus

c. Active sounds or passage of flatus

d. No bowel sounds, passage of flatus

48. All of the following are signs of urinary tract infection except:

a. Many white blood cells in the urine specimen

b. Edema in the lower extremities

c. Bacteria on culture

d. Burning on urination

49. Certain surgical procedures seem to create intense pain. An example of a surgical procedure that often causes intense pain is:

a. Rectal procedure

b. Hysterectomy

c. Ophthalmic procedure

d. Laminectomy

50. What is urinary retention?

a. Bladder fullness

b. Urgency

c. Absence of urination with suprapubic distention

d. Frequency

51. When is the most common occurrence of adynamic ileus?

a. After thoracic surgery

b. After cardiac surgery

c. After orthopedic surgery

d. After abdominal surgery

52. What paralyzes the smooth muscle of the bowel in adynamic ileus?

a. Low potassium levels

b. High potassium levels

c. Low phosphorus levels

d. High phosphorus levels

53. What is the treatment for adynamic ileus?

a. Increased fluid intake

b. Suspension of oral intake

c. Antibiotic therapy

d. Surgery

54. What causes postoperative pain?

a. Length of time in surgery

b. Fear and anxiety

c. Tissue damage

d. Injured nerve fibers

55. What type of drug can depress the respiratory effort?

a. Aspirin

b. Epileptic drugs

c. Narcotics

d. Insulin

56. Why would a patient complain of itching and rash after taking medication?

a. Overdose

b. Underdose

c. Drug allergy

d. To get attention

57. Postoperative pain is traditionally managed by:

a. Oral narcotics

b. Topical medications

c. Narcotic patches

d. Injection of narcotics

58. Inherent dangers of an epidural catheter include:

a. Hemorrhage and infection

b. Overmedication and infection

c. Undermedication and hemorrhage

d. Nausea and vomiting

59. The result of hemorrhage or infection of an epidural catheter is:

a. Respiratory arrest

b. Paraplegia

c. Itching and generalized rash

d. Adynamic ileus

60. What could be the result of medication drifting to higher levels in the spinal cord?

a. Paraplegia

b. Nausea and vomiting

c. Respiratory arrest

d. All of the above

61. On the pain intensity scale, a 5 would be:

a. No pain

b. Moderate pain

c. Worst possible

d. None of the above

62. The pain intensity scale rates pain from:

a. 0–10

b. 0–20

c. 0–5

d. 1–100

63. What is the purpose of the nasogastric tube?

a. To decrease nausea and vomiting

b. To keep the stomach evacuated

c. To keep the patient NPO

d. To prevent diarrhea

64. The normal amount of daily stomach secretions is:

a. 50–100 mL

b. 5–10 mL

c. 500–1000 mL

d. 1000–2000 mL

65. What would cause severe ear pain in a patient with a nasogastric tube?

a. Severe sore throat

b. Blocked bronchial tubes

c. Increased stomach secretions

d. Occluded eustachian tubes

66. The usual adult dose for aspirin is:

a. 650–975 mg every 4 hours

b. 550 mg initially followed by 275 mg every 4 hours

c. 1000 mg every 6 hours

d. 350–650 mg every 3 hours

67. The usual adult dose for naproxen (Naprosyn) is:

a. 650–975 mg every 8 hours

b. 1000–15000 mg twice a day

c. 500-mg initial dose followed by 250 mg every 6–8 hours

d. 50 mg every 4–6 hours

68. Terri Banks is a 5-year-old girl. She weighs 48 lb. What would the nurse expect the dose to be if the physician ordered acetaminophen?

a. 10 mg every 4 hours

b. 100–300 mg every 8 hours

c. 220–330 mg every 4 hours

d. 480–720 mg every 4 hours

69. The physician has ordered ibuprofen for Zack Hall, a 2-year-old who weighs 22 lb. What would an appropriate dose be for Zack?

a. 10 mg every 4 hours

b. 100 mg every 6–8 hours

c. 220 mg every 6 hours

d. 400 mg every 4–6 hours

70. What is the purpose of a dressing?

a. Provides a neat appearance

b. Provides a clean environment for the incision

c. Decreases pain in the postoperative phase

d. Reduces the chance of pulmonary complications

71. An appropriate use of a pressure dressing is in:

a. Carpal tunnel surgery

b. Cataract surgery

c. Thyroid surgery

d. Skin graft surgery

72. A chest tube, used to drain fluid from the lungs, would be removed:

a. When there is less than 200 mL of drainage in a day

b. When there is less than 500 mL of drainage in a day

c. When there is 10–30 mL of drainage in a day

d. When there is no drainage

73. How can one tell that the patient has an air leak when there is a chest tube in place?

a. The patient no longer coughs.

b. When the patient coughs, air bubbles appear in the water seal of the system.

c. There are no bubbles in the water seal when the patient coughs.

d. All patients have an air leak if the tube stays in for more than 6 days.

74. The most common reasons for failure of a closed drainage system are:

a. Improper tube size and skin breakdown

b. Improper placement and contamination

c. Loss of vacuum pressure and low pain threshold

d. Improper placement and loss of vacuum

75. When should the wound be redressed?

a. Every day

b. Every shift

c. When drainage is present or if the purpose of the dressing is to débride the wound

d. Not until discharge orders from the hospital have been written

✚ Answers

1. [a] On admission to the postanesthesia care unit (PACU)

Postoperative care begins when the patient is admitted to the PACU. (*page 229*)

2. [b] With the resolution of postoperative sequellae

Care after the operative or invasive procedure begins with admission of the patient to the PACU and ends with the resolution of postprocedure sequellae. (*page 229*)

3. [b] Drug allergies, type of surgery, pulmonary status

The report to PACU should include the patient's medical, social, and psychological history, such as chronic pulmonary disease, drug allergies, or a history of smoking. The type of procedure that was done and pertinent events that may have occurred during the procedure should also be described. (*page 229*)

4. [a] Several days

Massive tissue injury or the presence of foreign material intensifies inflammation. In a clean operative wound, inflammation lasts for several days. (*page 229*)

5. [b] 48 hours

Complete wound epithelialization usually has occurred within 48 hours. At this point, however, the wound is still weak. (*page 229*)

6. [c] 2–3 days

By the second or third day, the cellular phase begins. The fibrin strands that filled the wound in the inflammatory phase act as a framework for fibroblast invasion. Capillaries begin to proliferate to supply nutrients to the healing wound. (*page 229*)

7. [d] All phases

Protein deficiency delays almost every aspect of wound healing. Besides lowering the body's resistance to infection, protein deficiency, especially a prolonged deficiency, can cause massive tissue edema. (*page 230*)

8. [b] Vitamin K

Certain unsaturated fatty acids are essential to the inflammatory response, internal cell regulatory systems, and circulation. Vitamin K is essential for the synthesis of clotting factor. (*page 230*)

9. [a] Chemotherapeutic agents, anticoagulants

Some medications, such as corticosteroids and chemotherapeutic agents, inhibit wound healing. (*page 230*)

10. [d] Days 3–5

Signs of a urinary tract infection appear on the third to fifth postoperative day. (*page 231*)

11. [c] Chills and fever, skin warm to the touch

Infections manifest themselves in a variety of ways. However, the following signs of infection are always present: pain and tenderness due to irritation of local nerve endings, increased temperature of the area involved, and swelling due to edema and inflammatory exudate. (*page 231*)

12. [b] 24 hours

If the correct antibiotics are administered, the condition of the wound improves rapidly, usually within 24 hours. (*page 232*)

13. [d] Abscess

An abscess forms when the inflammatory process becomes suppurative, is confined within a single anatomical space, and is surrounded by granulation tissue. The abscess consists of purulent materials, necrotic host tissue, and bacteria. (*page 232*)

14. [a] Tender

An abscess is usually tender to the touch. If touched in this area, the patient most likely will indicate pain. (*page 232*)

15. [c] Drainage

The treatment of an abscess is drainage. Afterward, the physician can loosely pack the wound or insert a drain to keep it open and drained. (*page 232*)

16. [a] Impaired tissue integrity related to abscess formation

Risk factors associated with the nursing diagnosis *Risk for Impaired Tissue Integrity related to abscess formation* include presence of pus in the wound, inadequate wound drainage, and poor wound care. (*page 233*)

17. [c] *Risk for Impaired Tissue Integrity related to the formation of gas gangrene*

The risk factor associated with the nursing diagnosis *Risk for Impaired Tissue Integrity related to the formation of gas gangrene* is wound contamination with hemolytic streptococci or *Clostridium perfringens.* (*page 233*)

18. [d] *Risk for Impaired Skin Integrity: nonhealing wound*

Risk factors associated with the nursing diagnosis *Risk for Impaired Skin Integrity: nonhealing wound* include infection, hematomas, underlying diseases or conditions, adjacent tissue scarring or trauma, obesity, use of tape, and pressure from drain tubes. (*page 233*)

19. [a] *Risk for Alteration in Postoperative Cardiac Rate*

The risk factors associated with the nursing diagnosis *Risk for Alteration in Postoperative Cardiac Rate (tachycardia)* include fever, lack of medication routinely taken by the patient, relative hypotension, inadequate pain relief, and apprehension. (*page 234*)

20. [d] The patient smokes two packs of cigarettes a day

Risk factors associated with ineffective breathing patterns include stasis of pulmonary secretions, aspiration, smoking, and hypoventilation during anesthesia. (*page 234*)

21. [a] Postoperative urinary tract infection

Risk factors associated with postoperative urinary tract infection include dehydration, urinary retention, and indwelling urinary catheters. (*page 234*)

22. [c] Altered postprocedure bowel function

Risk factors associated with risk for altered postprocedure bowel function include manipulation of intestines during the procedure, decreased activity, narcotics, septicemia, hypovolemia, and hypokalemia. (*page 235*)

23. [d] Smoker

Risk factors associated with ineffective breathing patterns during the postprocedure period include stasis of pulmonary secretions, aspiration, smoking, hypoventilation during anesthesia, and handling of the pulmonary tissue during the procedure which leads to edema or alveolar damage. (*page 234*)

24. [d] Obese patient, surgical wound with undermined skin flap

Seromas are common in obese patients and in wounds with areas of undermined skin flaps. They consist of blood and protein-rich fluid. Seromas are usually sterile in the beginning but are susceptible to infections. (*page 235*)

25. [a] 20–35-mL syringe, 16-gauge needle, skin preparation solution

Supplies needed to aspirate a seroma include a 20–35-mL syringe, a 16–18-gauge needle, skin preparation solution, an adhesive bandage, and local anesthetic. (*page 236*)

26. [b] Two

Gas gangrene is caused by a combination of two processes: action of microbial enzymes in contact with healthy tissue and action of microbial enzymes indirectly through thrombosis of blood vessels supplying the tissue with nutrients. (*page 236*)

27. [c] Three

Several bacterial species, usually one aerobic and one anaerobic, cause synergistic gangrene. (*page 236*) There are three types of gas gangrene: aerobic, anaerobic, and synergistic. Extremely virulent strains of hemolytic streptococci usually cause aerobic gangrene. The gas bacillus *Clostridium perfringens* and related species cause anaerobic gangrene.

28. [b] 5th postoperative day

If it happens, wound dehiscence is most likely to appear on the 5th postoperative day. Infection is the precipitating factor in half of cases. Wound edge ischemia and wound closure under extreme tension are other causes of wound dehiscence. (*page 236*)

29. [c] Surgical closure

The treatment of choice for wound dehiscence or evisceration is surgical closure. (*page 236*)

30. [b] Supine

If evisceration occurs, measures to ensure the patient's safety must be implemented. The patient is placed in a supine position, and the wound is covered with sterile towels moistened with saline. Measures are taken to prevent hypovolemic shock. The patient is prepared for operative closure. (*page 236*)

31. [d] Transient low-grade

Elevated temperature can occur at any time after the procedure. Transient low-grade postprocedure fever, however, is considered normal. (*page 237*)

32. [c] Ambulation

Spiking temperatures during the first 2 days after the procedure are usually pulmonary in origin. The primary treatment is increased ambulation. (*page 237*)

33. [b] Pain and splinting

The major cause of ineffective cough is pain and splinting. Adequate pain relief can assist the patient in moving the secretions. How-ever, narcotics can depress respiratory function. (*page 238*)

34. [c] 2 days after the procedure

Pulmonary complications usually appear during the first 2 days after the procedure. These can involve atelectasis, infiltrate, or effusions. They are usually accompanied by an elevated temperature, tachycardia, restlessness, elevated white blood cell count, and lowered partial pressure of oxygen. (*page 238*)

35. [a] Bed rest

Segmental atelectasis can occur with bed rest or inadequate ventilation during an operative procedure. (*page 238*)

36. [a] Antibiotics

Pneumonia can develop as a result of massive or subtle aspiration. Sputum cultures may be positive. Antibiotics are included in treatment. (*page 238*)

37. [b] Pneumonia

Postprocedure pleural effusions can be caused by pneumonia, pulmonary embolus, congestive heart failure, or subdiaphragmatic abscess. (*page 238*)

38. [c] Fluid overload

Postoperative fluid overload can lead to congestive heart failure. It is characterized by vascular congestion and the inability of the heart to pump enough blood to meet the body's metabolic needs. (*page 238*)

39. [d] Congestive heart failure

Congestive heart failure is characterized by vascular congestion and the inability of the heart to pump enough blood to meet the body's metabolic needs. (*page 238*)

40. [b] Increased activity

The treatment for segmental atelectasis is to increase activity, such as ambulation. In some cases, incentive spirometry, postural drainage, percussion, inspiration of humidity, and tracheal suctioning may be used. In persistent cases, the patient may require therapeutic bronchoscopy. (*page 238*)

41. [a] Diuretics and inotropic drugs

Diuretics and inotropic drugs can be used in the treatment of overhydration. (*page 238*)

42. [b] Surgical and percutaneous drainage

Abscesses are readily seen with ultrasonography or computed tomography. The treatment is operative or percutaneous drainage of the abscess. (*page 238*)

43. [d] Prolonged venous cannulation, inactivity with venous stasis in the lower extremities

Thrombophlebitis results from inactivity, with venous stasis in the lower extremities as a complication of intravenous catheters. Prolonged venous cannulation or a chemical reaction from intravenous medications can cause thrombosis of a peripheral vein. (*page 238*)

44. [c] Deep veins of legs

By far the most serious form of thrombophlebitis occurs in the deep veins of the legs. (*page 238*)

45. [d] Application of elastic stockings, elevation of the legs

Thrombophlebitis can be prevented by maintaining high venous flow. This is accomplished by the application of elastic stockings, elevation of the legs, and muscular exercises. (*page 239*)

46. [a] Heparin

Heparin is the drug of choice for a patient with a diagnosis of thrombophlebitis. (*page 239*)

47. [c] Active sounds or passage of flatus

The first signs of returning bowel function include active bowel sounds and passage of flatus. If adynamic ileus is persistent, the nurse may suspect peritonitis, potassium depletion, or wound dehiscence. (*page 239*)

48. [b] Edema in the lower extremities

Signs of urinary tract infection include many white blood cells in the urine, bacteria on cultures, and burning on urination. Urine may be foul smelling or cloudy. (*page 239*)

49. [a] Rectal procedure

Severity of pain is related to the type of procedure. For example, knee and rectal procedures seem to create intense pain. (*page 240*)

50. [c] Absence of urination with suprapubic distention

Urinary retention is absence of urination with suprapubic distention. Measures to prevent urinary retention include activities that facilitate voiding, such as running water, assisting male patients in standing to void, and offering a bedpan or assistance to the bathroom every 2–3 hours. (*page 239*)

51. [d] After abdominal surgery

Adynamic ileus occurs most often after abdominal surgery. (*page 239*)

52. [a] Low potassium levels

Low serum potassium levels can paralyze the smooth muscles of the bowel in adynamic ileus. (*page 239*)

53. [b] Suspension of oral intake

The treatment for adynamic ileus is to withhold oral intake until bowel function returns. The patient may be relieved by the insertion of a nasogastric tube to evacuate the stomach contents. (*page 239*)

54. [d] Injured nerve fibers

Postoperative pain is caused by injured nerve fibers in the incised or traumatized tissue. The assessment of pain is an ongoing process that often begins as the patient returns to consciousness in the PACU. (*page 239*)

55. [c] Narcotics

A common side effect of narcotics is respiratory depression. An occasional patient exhibits a previously unknown allergy to the drug being used. (*page 240*)

56. [c] Drug allergy

The signs of a drug allergy are easily recognized by patient reports of itching and a generalized rash. The patient may also report tightness in the throat. Nausea and vomiting are also common side effects of narcotic use. (*page 240*)

57. [d] Injection of narcotics

Traditionally, acute pain is managed with intramuscular injections of narcotics. (*page 240*)

58. [a] Hemorrhage and infection

There are inherent dangers with the use of epidural catheters, such as hemorrhage and infection. (*page 240*)

59. [b] Paraplegia

If there is hemorrhage or infection around the epidural catheter, paraplegia can occur. (*page 240*)

60. [c] Respiratory arrest

If injected medication drifts to higher levels on the spinal cord, respiratory arrest can result. These patients must be closely monitored for complications while an epidural catheter is in place. (*page 240*)

61. [b] Moderate pain

A score of 5 on the pain intensity scale is considered moderate pain. (*page 241*)

62. [a] 0–10

The pain intensity scale rates pain on a scale of 0–10, where 0 indicates no pain and 10 indicates the worst possible pain. (*page 241*)

63. [b] To keep the stomach evacuated

The purpose of a nasogastric tube is to keep the stomach evacuated. It is used to treat nausea and vomiting with distention from the ileus. (*page 242*)

64. [c] 500–1000 mL

Normally, the stomach secretes 500–1000 mL/day. (*page 242*)

65. [d] Occluded eustachian tubes

Severe ear pain can indicate acute otitis media if the nasogastric tube occludes the eustachian tube. (*page 243*)

66. [a] 650–975 mg every 4 hours

The usual adult dose of aspirin is 650–975 mg every 4 hours. (*page 243*)

67. [c] 500-mg initial dose followed by 250 mg every 6–8 hours

The usual adult dose for naproxen is 500-mg initial dose followed by 250 mg every 6–8 hours. (*page 243*)

68. [c] 220–330 mg every 4 hours

48 lb = 22 kg: Take 22 kg × 10 = 220 and 22 kg × 15 = 330. Your answer is 220–330 mg every 4 hours. (*page 243*)

69. [b] 100 mg every 6–8 hours

22 lb = 10 kg: 10 kg × 10 mg = 100 mg. Your answer is 100 mg every 6–8 hours. (*page 243*)

70. [b] Provides a clean environment for the incision

The purpose of dressings is to provide a clean environment for the incision, preventing the introduction of pathogens into the wound before the wound edges can seal. Wound edges seal to bacteria within 4 hours. (*page 243*)

71. [d] Skin graft surgery

One appropriate use of pressure dressing is on skin grafts. Pressure ensures that the donor skin stays in contact with the blood supply at the graft site. (*page 243*)

72. [a] When there is less than 200 mL of drainage in a day

The decision to remove the chest tube depends on its function. If its purpose is to drain fluid and superlative exudate, it can be removed when less than 200 mL/day is draining from the chest. If its purpose is to evacuate air, it can be removed when there is no evidence of an air leak. (*page 244*)

73. [b] When the patient coughs, air bubbles appear in the water seal of the system.

An air leak is present if air bubbles appear in the water seal of the system when the patient coughs. (*page 244*)

74. [d] Improper placement and contamination

The most common reasons for failure of a closed drainage system include inadequate diameter of the tube, improper placement or displacement of tube, loss of vacuum pressure, occlusion of the drain fenestration with clot or tissue, and retrograde contamination of the wound during emptying. (*page 244*)

75. [c] When drainage is present or if the purpose of the dressing is to débride the wound

The wound should be redressed only when drainage is present or if the purpose of the dressing is to débride the wound. (*page 245*)